Crossing the Moon

Crossing the Moon

A Journey Through Infertility

•

PAULETTE BATES ALDEN

Hungry Mind Press
Saint Paul · Minnesota

Published by Hungry Mind Press
57 Macalester Street
Saint Paul, Minnesota 55105

Publishers note:
Portions of this work were originally published, in somewhat
different form, in the *New York Times Magazine* and
Ploughshares.

With the exceptions of family members, famous people, and
Dr. Kuneck and his staff, the author has changed the names in
this book.

9 8 7 6 5 4 3 2 1
First Hungry Mind Press printing, 1996

Library of Congress Catalog Card Number: 96-76411
ISBN 1-886913-08-0

Printed in the United States of America

Jacket Design: Julie Metz
Cover Photographs: © Barry Marcus
Book Design: Will H. Powers
Typesetting: Stanton Publication Services, Inc.

For my mother
Marie Southerlin Bates

and in loving memory of my father
Paul Goodlett Bates

Acknowledgments

This book has been a long labor, and many people have helped me along the way. Special thanks to Phillip Lopate who read an early draft of the manuscript and offered invaluable criticism when he was the Loft's 1992 Creative Non-fiction Writer-in-Residence. Thanks, too, to my fellow students in that workshop, all talented writers, who gave me generous support and suggestions: Peter Carlton, Shawn Gillen, Jim Goralski, Nancy Meyer, and Melanie Richards. My heartfelt gratitude goes out to all those who either read the manuscript in progress or offered help in other ways: my sister, Betty Bates; Dale Davis, for her constant belief in me; Sandra Benítez; Rebecca Biderman; Blanche McCrary Boyd; Jill Breckenridge; Marisha Chamberlain; Beverly Donofrio; Mary Kay Herr; Mary Junge; Vicky Lettmann; Valerie Miner; Jane McDonnell; Sheila Murphy; Mary Petrie; Louise Ritzmann Roche; Mary Rockcastle; Clare Rossini; Madelon Sprengnether; Susan Allen Toth; Annette Turow; Susan Welch; and Al Young.

I also want to thank the folks at Hungry Mind Press for bringing this book into the world: Page

Cowles, Pearl Kilbride, Gail See, David Unowsky, and especially Margaret Wurtele, for calling back. I'm very grateful to Brigitte Frase for her sound editorial advice, to Mary Dupont for all her good help in the office, and to Mary Byers for her excellent copyediting. I owe a special debt of gratitude to John and Meredith Alden, for their constant support and love. Thanks to the Ragdale Foundation in Lake Forest, Illinois, for putting me up and leaving me alone to write. And thanks to everyone who has ever said a kind word to me about my writing.

And thank you, Jeff, for reading the Dairy Queen scene more times than anyone would believe and for crossing every moon with me.

I

1

It's an unseasonably warm afternoon in April, 1986, and I'm sitting on a stone bench outside a Dairy Queen near our house in Minneapolis, considering the two mothers and three children who share my table. I'm about to turn thirty-nine years old, which is why I'm so interested in mothers and children.

I haven't always been so interested. In fact, for most of my adult life I've behaved as if mothers and children had nothing to do with me, which, on the whole, they haven't. But lately I can't take my eyes off them. I'm in the process of making (for me) a mind-boggling discovery: women have children. It's what women *do*. A lot of them, it seems. Most of them, from what I can tell. Now that the blinders have dropped from my eyes, I'm amazed, dazzled, puzzled, and afraid.

One of the mothers is younger than I, the first detail I note about her. Blond hair, good teeth, and I wonder if she works outside the home, since it's the middle of the afternoon and she's in Bermuda shorts. For all I know she's the president of IBM, but something tells me her job is raising the little girl beside her who is eating an ice cream cone dipped in waxy-looking butterscotch. The ice cream is running down the child's hands, grasped around the cone in a double-fisted grip, dripping onto her shorts and bare legs, which are covered in downy hair so fair it is translucent. There is a pasty white ring around her mouth, which I would love to wipe off. The mother has a handful of cheap paper napkins, which she's going through in a desultory way — she's been to Dairy Queen before — while issuing a soft series of admonitions I seem vaguely to remember from my own childhood: "Why don't you lick around the cone to keep it from dripping? . . . here . . . let me help you . . . won't you let me hold it for you? . . . oh, Sarah! . . . now look what you've done!"

I try to imagine these mother-words issuing from my own lips. I can't imagine keeping up the constant murmuring that motherhood requires. But I have felt how my hand, of its own volition, wanted to reach out and wipe that child's mouth.

The other mother at the table is actually as old as I, but of course she already has her children. We arrived in the parking lot at the same time. I simply got out of my car and went in. While I waited in line, I watched this mother get out, go around to the trunk, get the stroller out, open it, lift the baby into it, buckle him in, help the other child, a boy about three, out of the car, push the stroller to the glass door, open it, maneuver the stroller into the crowded space while trying to keep track of her little boy, who made a beeline for the condiments bar, where he happily began fishing dill pickle slices out with his fingers.

I felt dizzy with relief that I was not a mother. I got my hamburger wrapped in gold foil and hurried out to sit in the sun, tired, hungry, and wild to be alone.

But the only spot available was at the table with the young blond mother and little girl. And then when the older mother had her order, she pushed the stroller out the glass door and looked around for a place to sit. Naturally she pushed it right up next to me. And in spite of myself, I smiled and moved over to make room.

By now the little girl has ice cream pretty much all over her. "Oh well, I'll just have to throw her in the bathtub when I get home anyway," the younger mother says, and laughs self-deprecatingly, as if the joke were on her. I am touched by her—to say the mundane, the unremarkable thing. The two mothers begin conversing, exchanging information about the children's ages and such, but what I want to know is, *What is it like to be a mother?* I want the skinny, the good and the bad, the sublime and the tedious.

But it's a warm spring afternoon at Dairy Queen and I'm not about to rend the social fabric by asking such a question. Besides, I know what they'd probably say, once they recovered from the shock of someone so out of it. They might start with a little humor, but then if I pressed them on it, go on to say that children change your life, but that they are worth it. Which doesn't really speak to the uninitiated. So what I must really want to know is something neither they nor anyone else can tell me: Should *I* be a mother?

I had a Little Ricky doll when I was ten years old. He was the son of Lucy and Ricky Ricardo, and I loved him intensely the summer our family took a Western trip in our '57 Chevy station wagon. I gave him his little bottle, changed his clothes out of his own little suitcase, showed him the passing cacti and red rock mesas out the window, made sure he got his naps, tucked him in in our motel room at night. The first thing I thought of in the morning was Ricky—his round plastic face, his hard blue crystal eyes that blinked open, his shapely limbs, like pale link sausages, his pleasingly plump torso, his intoxicating rubber smell. He completely filled my senses. The sight, the smell, the feel of him gave me deep pleasure. All I wanted or needed—then—was Ricky.

Still, I remember how relieved I was when I moved on to plastic horses. Cathy Meyers from up the road had a black stallion and I had a buckskin one, and we'd race them for hours across the wide-open expanse of our basement floors. The horses were always having to escape captivity, a plot we never tired of, until we discovered boys. We were twelve by then, going on thirteen, and perhaps we sensed what was waiting for us up ahead. It would have nothing to do with wild horses.

I ponder the three children at our table, lost as they are in their revelry of cold sweet cream. In a way they're adorable, and then again, just the usual young of the species. I try to imagine what it would be like if I had a little child, if I had brought him or her to Dairy Queen today.

About the closest I can come to imagining what it would be like to have a child is with our cat, Cecil. For Cecil I feel the most delicious love, but also the most anxious responsibility. My husband, Jeff, loves Cecil too, but he can go to sleep at night if Cecil isn't in. I have to get up every fifteen minutes or so to check for him. When he finally does appear, I sweep him up in my arms, burying my nose in his cold fur that smells of our neighbor's arborvitae bush. He's always on my mind, even when I'm not thinking about him.

How much worse would it be with a child? How much worse, that is, would *I* be? I'm not sure I want to unleash all that maternal instinct. Would I ever feel free again? Would I ever be *alone*? I don't just mean by myself; it isn't as if I haven't heard of babysitters. I know that other women do it—have selves and babies, too. But I'm not sure I can be one of them. I remember Ricky-love.

The children, having finished their ice cream, have begun a game of chase around our table, catching onto their mothers' hips as round and round they go. The baby in the stroller regards these antics with wide-eyed amazement, as if seeing such a sight for the first time, which perhaps he is. But suddenly the little boy trips and falls, and after a moment of stunned silence in which he checks himself over to see if he's okay, lets out a bawl. We three women rise as one, but his mother is there first, hoisting him whimpering into her arms: "Does it hurt? Mama make it better," and she kisses the tiny finger he holds out, sweetly, to her lips.

And before I can stop it, I'm filled with a sudden anguish: *I might never have a child!* A grief worthy of a death wells in me, before there has even been a life. *I might never have a child*, and the irony is not lost on me, that I'm not even sure I want one. And alongside that is another shape just coming into focus, which I don't want to see, but which is drawing closer every day: I might not be able to. It might already be too late, I might already be too old, there might be something wrong.

It's true that Jeff and I are not using birth control. We haven't been for quite some time (I won't let myself remember how long). But I tell myself we're not really *trying*. Trying is for people who want a child, and I'm not sure. Jeff is leaving it mainly up to me. He says he can be happy either way, and besides, he has his hands full, dealing with the barely contained insanity of a small law firm, something they didn't teach him in law school. We both know it would be my life that would change the most if we had a child. Maybe it doesn't have to be that way, but that's the way it is. Jeff would still get dressed in a suit every day, and go off to his office downtown, and I would be mainly responsible for baby.

I believe in making a conscious choice where having a child is concerned. But in the meantime, I've been hoping nature would just take its course. But nothing has ever happened. I haven't gotten pregnant. I'm not going to be let off the hook. If we do want a child, if we're ever going to have one, we've got to do something about it.

The little boy has joined the little girl, who is now prying pebbles out of the rocky soil at the edge of the cement patio. And now the younger blond mother stands up, smooths her Bermuda shorts, and calls to the little girl that it is time to go. But the little girl has other plans. "Don't want to go," she whines. "But we have to go home and make dinner for Daddy," her mother reasons nicely, offering her hand, which the little girl refuses to take. She eyes the little boy sadly, with what might be the first stirrings of lust. "No," she insists, "don't want to go. I wanna play!" And she throws herself down, crying, on some grass, brown and defeated after our long Minnesota winter. The two mothers give each other a long-suffering look, while an exasperated snort breaks through the blond mother's lips.

"We're going to go *now*," she says, an edge in her

voice. This can only go on for so long. And still the child screams and kicks. The terrible, the *terrible* twos! Or is she three?

Finally the mother snatches her up by the arm. "This is completely unnecessary," she says in a no-nonsense voice. "You stop it right now!" The girl screams louder.

Could you ever just leave a child at Dairy Queen? Just pretend it wasn't yours and get in your car and drive away?

The baby in the stroller is regarding me with inscrutable dark blue eyes. He offers no expression, nor do I, staring back, controlling my face muscles, which long to lapse into some silly expression suitable for coaxing a smile from an infant. He's dressed in a baby outfit—a sailor suit and middy blouse. His feet are bare. I study the tiny toes. I feel the impulse rise in me to exclaim something in a high female voice, such as "What darling little feet! Just look at those tiny toes!" while my hand practices its part in my imagination, reaching out to touch them. But just as quickly another part of me reaches out and swats that hand.

I wad my foil into a gold ball and toss it into the trash can that Dairy Queen has so optimistically provided. When I get to my car, I turn and look back at the mothers. They're on mother-time, or maybe it's kid-time, but whatever it is it isn't my time. I start my old Honda and in a few minutes I'm home, pushing the electric garage door opener, watching with pleasure as the door actually opens. I don't take it for granted that we have an electric garage door opener, a garage to open, two more or less reliable cars to put in it, and a house we're buying, to boot. I'm still getting used to this house, even though we've lived in it for several years. When we were first house hunting, I kept looking for something Southern, not easy to find in Minnesota. The closest we came was an old farmhouse built around the turn of the century, but the door frames were so askew none of the doors would shut properly. We settled for Minnesota plumb, this solid-looking stucco house built to withstand the harsh winters and looking that way to me. It still surprises me that I've ended up here, in the Midwest, the middle, but maybe it's fitting somehow, halfway between the two great poles of my life, my South Carolina girlhood of white gloves and panty girdles, and my California twenties of free love and consciousness-raising.

I come in through the backyard, over the sunken concrete blocks that serve as a walkway, inspecting the side garden for any new shoots. Spring has arrived with such suddenness that I see bulb tips pushing through the ground that weren't there when I left a few hours ago. I unlock the back door, balancing a bag of groceries on my hip, and let myself in. The house is quiet, but as soon as he hears me, Cecil comes stretching from whatever soft spot he was sleeping on. I make my voice into a little song, stroking him with sound as I carry the groceries into the kitchen.

I put away oatmeal and Triscuits, and turn on the TV on top of the refrigerator, hoping for Oprah. I love Oprah, a detail I never mention to my colleagues, as they like to refer to themselves, in the English department at the university. I teach creative writing part-time, a lowly adjunct, but it gives me time to write. Today's show is on mothers who married their daughters' boyfriends. I put away soup, lettuce, chicken. I keep hoping she'll do a show on aging women who can't make up their minds about motherhood.

I want to look something up. I go upstairs to my study, Cecil bounding before me. I get out my old copy of *Of Woman Born*. The dust jacket is yellow with age, and it smells of mildew. I look up the copyright date: 1976. I was twenty-nine years old then, single, trying to reinvent myself from books like this one. I carried it to Tacoma, Washington, when I moved there with Jeff, and I brought it back here when we returned, married, in 1980. I moved it from our first rental house to our second rental house to this house we're buying now.

It's underlined throughout, and I've made notes in the margins. The first sign of my own response comes in the preface and is, appropriately enough, a question mark by the line, "We know more about the air we breathe, about the seas we travel, than

about the nature and meaning of motherhood."
Then I really got down to underlining. "I only knew
that I had lived through something which was considered central to the lives of women, fulfilling even
in its sorrow, a key to the meaning of life; and that
I could remember little except anxiety, physical
weariness, anger, self-blame, boredom, and dividing
within myself."

All the things I've wanted to avoid.

I look over at my desk. I got up at six-thirty this
morning to be at that desk by eight. I was very
sleepy, so I began by reading a short story in *The
New Yorker*. Then I turned to a story of my own,
which I had started a few weeks ago. I began to see
the story not as a linear thing, but as a sphere. Still,
it was hard work, tiring, and by eleven I felt exhausted. But I pushed on, writing some sketchy sentences that might be good—someday—not now—
and finally let myself off the hook by typing up the
good story from *The New Yorker*. I studied the sentences as I typed, how each one was clear and per-
ceptive, how each did more than one thing. Often
lately when I'm working, I'm aware, dimly and
brightly, not wanting to call too much attention to
it, that yes, this is it, this is writing, I'm making some
progress, I'm doing it.

Would I still be able to do that if I had a baby?
Would I even want to?

I have thought about it, and I can honestly say
that I have never seen my mother sitting at a desk,

writing. I have seen her do many useful things, but never that. She's always busy, thinking up more and more things that need to be done, and when she finally does sit down in the evenings, it is to watch TV.

My mother is sitting in the car, waiting, while my sister and I have our piano lessons. Inside, belaboring the Moonlight Sonata, my sister and I imagine ourselves playing concerts at Carnegie Hall, or more modestly, at the very least, being the piano teacher—Mrs. Young, with her coffee breath and her connection to greatness: she has busts of Beethoven and Brahms on her Steinway. Meanwhile, out in the car, our mother, who once played piano herself, who even gave lessons before WE were born, sits reading a magazine. Waiting.

It's just that lately I've found myself browsing in the parenting and childbirth sections of bookstores, reading up on fertility with the same covert feelings I had as a teenager when I sneaked a look at books on sex. I feel there is something unseemly in an almost thirty-nine-year-old woman boning up on fertility. Finally I bought a book called *Fertility Awareness*. When I took it to the checkout counter, I held it close to my chest so no one could see the title.

I reshelve *Of Woman Born* next to *Fertility Awareness*. According to *Fertility Awareness*, cervical mucus is a good indicator of approaching ovulation. A year ago I didn't even know I had cervical mucus, and now I'm an expert on it. I go in the bathroom and read the sign: there is a stringy clear blob of the stuff, which stretches into a long shiny thread, my most fertile time.

When Jeff comes home from work I follow him upstairs to talk while he changes his clothes.

"Work was the usual maelstrom," Jeff says as he takes off his tie. "You know the new woman associate we hired? The one who came from that big New York firm? She quit. Just like that. No notice, no new job, nothing. When she walked out the door, I felt like following her."

"Maybe you should quit," I say, not for the first time.

"And then what? I have to hang in there, get the experience." He is taking off his blue oxford cloth shirt, stained under the arms. Being a lawyer makes him sweat. "So how was your day?"

"Fine, okay," I say slowly. "But guess what. I have that kind of mucus I read about."

"Spit?"

"Spin."

"I thought you didn't want a child."

"I don't. And I probably can't get pregnant anyway. It's just that I've got this fantastic mucus . . . it seems a shame to waste it."

Jeff turns and grins at me. He is in his plaid boxer shorts. "Do we have to do it right now? I was hoping for a drink."

"Oh, I don't know," I say and grimace. "But maybe we should jump on it." I look at Jeff's body. He has a

wonderfully hairy chest, nice legs, and great big
hands and feet. He is entirely pleasing to me, a fact
that never ceases to amaze me. In my vast and var-
ied experience prior to Jeff, I ran across a lot of
things in men that didn't suit me.

"So you're going to make a big deal over this,"
he says, sitting down beside me on the bed. "First
woman in the history of the world to get pregnant."
He lays me back sideways on the bed. "Does this
mean we're now *trying*?"

"It is a big deal. It'll change our lives forever if it
happens. And no, this is not really trying. This is still
not-trying."

"We're ready for a little change. Change won't
hurt us a bit." He is sliding off my shorts, slipping off
my T-shirt.

"A little change," I mutter. "A little change, *he*
says."

We are tussling around on the bed a bit.

"I bet we score."

"Oh, great, a sports metaphor. Listen," I say, "I
thought a kid should be conceived in passion."

"This is passion."

"This is a lot of fooling around."

"Don't talk," Jeff says. "Don't talk."

2

So how was it, I wondered, that I had arrived at this point in my life: almost thirty-nine years old, no child? When I looked back, I could see why, and even when, I took a sharp turn away from motherhood. I could also see why motherhood would catch up with me.

I was raised to be a virgin until I married. Not that anyone ever said this to me directly. Such a general truth didn't need to be spelled out. It never seriously crossed my mind, in high school, to go all the way. I had boyfriends with whom I made out, madly, but I was saving myself for marriage. For a girl like me, virginity was the Big Given, the monumental monolithic Given from which all the other givens sprang. The whole social structure balanced delicately on that thin membrane. If I couldn't have sex until marriage, that dictated quite nicely that I would marry, sooner rather than later no doubt, and that I would be a wife, and as night follows day, a mother. *Virgin-wife-mother*. It was all I knew, and all I needed to know.

I had a boyfriend my sophomore year of college who wanted to marry me. After we graduated, of course. We were both enrolled in small private schools in North Carolina, his for boys, mine for girls (we were not yet men and women). Unlike me, Bill already knew what he wanted to be: an orthopedic surgeon. His father was an orthopedic surgeon. We sort of assumed I would be a high school English teacher, if I had to be anything at all.

What Bill and I had in common, besides our profound youth, was a great desire to please our parents. My parents loved Bill Nelson. He was everything they hoped for in a future son-in-law. I loved Bill Nelson — at least I thought I did. I loved it that he matched my parents' expectations, which I still assumed were my own. I was highly sensitive to what my parents and, by extension, society expected of me. I was well aware of what was valued, acceptable, respectable, approved. Bill fit the bill.

The moment came, however, when I threw it all over. This was the moment when I began to turn away from motherhood, though I didn't know it at the time. I just thought I was dumping Bill. In a way it was like one of those Frankenstein monster stories, where a previously inanimate form springs to life and takes over. This was the moment when my real self made herself known, and her first word was "no."

The breath of life, the spark that ignited this dormant self was Bill's parents' French Provincial living room furniture. We were driving somewhere in Bill's little white Skylark convertible (there was a plastic rose on the antenna, a romantic touch). Bill was telling me how his parents were going to give us their French Provincial living room furniture when we got married. I had never seen this furniture, and so he described it to me in detail—the curved legs of the sofa and chairs, the cool blue of the upholstery, the pale coffee table. I'm sure it was quite nice. A vision came into my mind, of Bill and me lounging around on his parents' French Provincial living room furniture in our future married life. This was supposed to be a beautiful scenario for a girl like me.

But suddenly, I didn't want it. I didn't want it at all! I didn't want his parents' French Provincial living room furniture, I didn't want married bliss, and most of all, I didn't want Bill.

Nothing had ever been so clear to me. I couldn't wait to get away from him. I almost jumped out of the car. Of course I rode on, demurely, but in my heart I was already gone.

It took several weeks to break up with him. After all, nothing really had happened; it wasn't anything he *did*. It was hard on my parents. I couldn't explain, when my parents, teary-eyed, asked me why I didn't love Bill anymore. I just didn't. In fact, I could hardly stand to be around him, though out of common decency I made myself pretend he wasn't loathsome to me. I was shocked at myself, but there was no getting around what I really felt: I couldn't wait for the day when Bill—and all he represented—would be out of my life forever.

I told my parents that I wanted to transfer to the University of North Carolina, because it had a writing program. I harbored a secret dream of becoming a writer, so secret, in fact, I could barely acknowledge it to myself. Girls like me didn't become writers; they became wives and mothers. But at that moment in Bill's car, I had seen clearly that if I married Bill, if I became a wife and mother, I would never be a writer.

I had first visited Chapel Hill the spring of my freshman year, when the girls at our college filled out questionnaires for a fee and were matched with boys at neighboring schools. My date at Chapel Hill had been an intense young man, a philosophy major, with beautiful dark hair and eyes, quite a bit on the ethereal side. I found him irresistible, which he did not find me, but he was nice to me and showed me around. I had not known that there were places big enough in the world to lose oneself, to become anonymous. I was used to everyone knowing my business, which, I now began to sense uneasily, was rapidly coming to be to lose my virginity. I sensed, like the tadpole, that I was about to transmogrify, and I wanted a pond big enough to do it in. I felt strange twitchings in my extremities, odd internal pushings.

The first thing I did when I got to Chapel Hill was sign up for a creative-writing course. The teacher, Max Steele, was from my hometown, Greenville,

South Carolina. I hadn't known that writers could come from Greenville. I didn't know much about writers, never having met one.

I did know, however, that writers were not virgins. Writers were everything that was not *virgin-wife-mother*.

Of course losing my virginity was no easy matter for me. I'm sure there were plenty of young men at Chapel Hill who would have been pleased to relieve me of my burden, but I was not about to lay aside lightly the most fundamental tenet of my life. I had the additional problem of equating sex not with love or passion, but with morality. I had been raised Southern Baptist, after all.

I spent my first fall at Chapel Hill reading about situation ethics and the new morality. Still, more and more often, I found myself in strange scenes with a changing cast of boys. Despite the various settings, these situations had in common someone's hand down someone's pants. Still, I wrestled with my virginity like B'rer Rabbit with Tar Baby.

Once I almost did it, almost gave myself to an art student who had taken me out in the woods near a dam in the country. At the last moment he confessed he had a girlfriend. How shaken I had been! I had almost done the wrong thing with the wrong person at the wrong time for the wrong reasons. Still, it would have been a relief to have it over with, once and for all.

At the end of the school year, I didn't go home

for the summer, but stayed on campus, ostensibly to take a course. When the Southern summer rolled in, like a big wave, knocking everyone over, I took to spreading myself out on the hard concrete by the campus pool. I gave myself up to Fate, and soon enough, along it came in a pair of thin, white gym shorts.

The first view I had of destiny was a very hairy leg right beside my face when I opened my eyes after falling asleep one particularly hot day by the pool. For a moment I thought I was seeing not a person's leg at all, but that of some strange animal I couldn't identify. The man to whom this leg belonged stooped down beside me, breathing very hard, and sweating: his musky odor penetrated even the chlorine air around the pool. When finally I looked in his face, I saw big white teeth grinning at me, like the wolf in *Little Red Riding Hood*, all interest and appetite.

Beside the pool the man's white German shepherd was crouched down on his front legs, his hindquarters raised indelicately in the air, lapping the chlorine water. I had seen the two of them often, the man and the dog, moving across campus with the same motions. I had never seen the dog go to other people, like normal friendly dogs, or bother with other animals, for that matter. He was always loping along with his nose close to the ground, as if he was searching for something, and everything else was just in the way.

"I've seen you around," the man said, and he grinned at me with his big white teeth.

I was surprised. That anyone—that he—should have noticed me. But maybe it was the bohemian clothes I had started to wear, black tops and Indian print skirts. It was easy to look bohemian when all the other coeds wore Villager shirtwaists and Weejuns. At the beginning of the summer I had taken an apartment by myself. It was 1968, the first year the university would allow girls to live off campus. That made me something of a bohemian, too. Anything to separate myself from the sticky mass of Southern girls who clung together like honey bees in the dorm.

"Hey, Wolfgang! Here!" the man called, and the dog came loping to where he stooped. I tried to pet him, but he moved away from me and regarded me with his yellow neutral eyes.

"I'm afraid he's not the friendly sort," the man said, burying his fingers deep in the stiff white fur. "Why don't you have dinner with me tonight?"

My mind went into action, processing a polite excuse. Instead, I said, "Why not?" surprising myself.

"Good!" the man said. "Good! Good!"

His name was Joel Goldetski, and his occupation, campus politico. He was twenty-six years old, Jewish, had sinus trouble, and had dropped out of graduate school in political science to agitate. All this he told me in a great laughing way, but I had trouble getting the joke, fearing it was on me. He was dark where I was fair, masculine where I was feminine, Northern where I was Southern. He drove a beat-up old Lincoln full of white dog hair and books, and in the back seat I noticed a ratty blanket, full of significance. He didn't help me with my door.

We drove to his place because he wanted to take a shower. It was a basement apartment in a row of cheap concrete block buildings of washed-out pastels. There was a mattress on the floor, books piled everywhere, and one poster on the wall, of Lenin.

When Joel emerged from the bathroom, he was wearing another pair of shorts, hardly anything at all. For dinner he fixed a cheese omelette, and we drank cheap bittersweet wine out of coffee mugs. I had never met anyone who talked like Joel. It wasn't just his accent. It was his *words*. There were so many of them, all nasal and Northern and fast. I could hardly follow the sense of things, but it didn't seem to matter. I couldn't take my mind off his big white teeth.

When eventually we found ourselves in bed, and I, naked, waxed uncertain, Joel didn't try to persuade me. He said it was up to me. He got up to take another shower, leaving me alone in bed with the sound of water running. I was used to a little more in the way of pressure; the lack of drama was a letdown. When Joel got back in bed, he had on striped pajamas and began to read the newspaper. He wore black-rimmed glasses to read. After he finished the editorials, he turned out the light, climbed on top of me, and we did it.

I tried to stay awake to record the momentous event in my memory. But actually, there had been very little to remember. Cars were going by above our heads on the street, and occasionally the beams would flash through like searchlights. I wondered if my landlady would realize I hadn't come in that night. She would *know*. I fell asleep with the thought that I had changed my life.

Sometime in the night, I woke with a terrible start and sat straight up in bed. First I was aware of being afraid, then I remembered where I was, and then I remembered the dream. My parents had driven from my hometown in South Carolina to the university. They had known exactly where to find me, and they had burst into Joel's room. The dream gave me a sick feeling. Beside me Joel was snoring in an ungodly fashion. Maybe he would expire, and I would be left to explain to the police. When I couldn't stand it another moment, I reached over and turned his head to the other side, away from me. I couldn't get back to sleep. I imagined roaches crawling on the cement walls. It was odd to be lying so close to the floor; Joel was not into creature comforts. I stared into the darkness, wondering if I had ruined my life. Maybe I would get lice.

But in the light of day, I was in love. I liked everything about Joel, even the hair in his nose. He was my first lover, which, I told myself, was romantic in and of itself. We went out to breakfast at the Pineroom. It had dark wooden booths, played classical music, and the people who went there smoked pipes, wore beards, and played chess. I felt very adult, having scrambled eggs in public the morning after I'd spent the whole night in bed with a man. Joel was older and darker than anyone I knew. I looked back with disdain on the little blond Southern boys on whose fraternity beds I had wiggled in girlish indecision. I had left them in the dust.

I contemplated how suddenly, overnight, everything had changed. The previous year, when I had lived in a dorm, my best friend, Susan Alexander, and I had sat for hours cross-legged on our twin beds, talking across the linoleum about what to do about our virginity. Susan's father, a Baptist minister, had told her if she slept with a man before marriage, she would be making The Ultimate Statement. Susan had a round child's face, a cap of golden hair, and great big breasts like a fertility goddess. She had fallen in love with a graduate student in English, but it scared her to make The Ultimate Statement, so at the end of the school year, when I had gotten my efficiency apartment, Susan had gotten married. That summer we had seen very little of each other. Faced with a similar problem, we had found different solutions, and each wondered if *she* were the fool.

There was the question of contraceptives. I certainly didn't want to get pregnant. Babies before marriage ruined if not your life then certainly your reputation, possibly more important.

Joel would pull out at the crucial time but that was nerve-wracking. I understood that I was supposed to be responsible for not getting pregnant. I made an appointment at the campus infirmary. I debated whether to make up a story about being engaged. It was not for nothing that I had had an ethics course. I knew in the same way I knew I was supposed to wait until marriage that the infirmary wouldn't give the pill to unmarried girls.

I was shown into a Dr. Schur's office. I had to wait a long time. Lately my nerves had felt stretched, like rubber bands about to pop. There had been the uncomfortable business of my landlady always peeping out the window when I came wheeling my mother's old Buick into the yard in the morning, staying only long enough to change clothes. Prior to Joel, I had been on the best of terms with her, the perfect virgin daughter. Now she never came out when I was there. I had no idea if that was on purpose, or just circumstantial. I had lost the perspective of the straight road, having stepped off onto the shoulder, gone down the bank, and entered the dark forest.

Dr. Schur came in and shook my cold hand. "Now, what can I do for you?" he asked, taking his seat behind the desk. He had on a white coat that matched his white hair. He was old enough to be Father Time.

"I'd like to go on the pill," I said in a tiny voice.

He gave me a benevolent smile. Everybody loves a bride. "I see. Are you engaged, then, my dear?" He was making a notation in my folder.

"No, sir."

"I see. Bad cramps, maybe?"

"No, sir. It's just that I . . . I . . . I . . ." I couldn't think exactly how to word it. "I'm having intercourse, and I need a contraceptive." I blushed so deeply the top of my head tingled.

He stopped writing and eyed me for a long time across the polished wood, contemplatively, as if he had just now noticed me. "I see," he said at last, though I wasn't sure he saw at all. Absentmindedly I checked the buttons on my blouse to make sure they were buttoned. "As you must know," he said, "this university has a policy against giving the pill to unmarried girls. It just isn't done. I imagine in a few years—by 1970 even—it will be routine. But for now that's the policy, and I'm required to go along with it." He paused thoughtfully. "I'm sure many girls who come in here make up a story about getting married, and then we do help them. If you see what I mean."

We both sat in silence while I thought this over.

"Well, thanks anyway," I said, my throat aching. I fell into a deep study of my skirt.

"Do you mind telling me why you chose not to?"

It was hard to find the words. My voice halted. "Because if I lied it would make what I'm doing seem wrong. And I don't believe it is wrong. I can't explain it very well."

"I think you explain it very well," Dr. Schur said. He leaned back in his chair, fingertips one on one. "I respect your position. It shows integrity."

My hand quivered in my lap.

"I can give you the name of a doctor in town," he said, "who might be able to help you out. I don't know how he feels about these things, but he's a good man. And I wish you luck." Then he stood and shook my hand.

Joel was waiting for me in the Pineroom. When I sat down, I couldn't help beaming. I held up the piece of paper.

"Ah," Joel said. "The prescription."

"As good as. It's the name of a doctor in town who can fix me up. The infirmary won't give pills to unmarried girls."

"Sometimes I forget about the South," Joel sighed. "Until you remind me."

I didn't quite understand what he meant. I had hardly been out of the Carolinas, and then mainly with my family on trips to visit relatives in Texas. Philadelphia, which was where Joel was from, might have been another planet. Joel spoke differently from me; he acted differently. I liked to think of him as a dark, romantic stranger, but sometimes, such as when he blew his nose, he didn't seem quite romantic enough. And besides, he never told me he loved me and something in me kept waiting. Sometimes he acted too much like an older brother. He stood on the sidelines and waved encouragement to me, but beyond that, he didn't help me. He wouldn't carry the ball of my life, no matter how often I indicated to him that I wanted to toss it his way.

I made an appointment with the doctor in town. The nurse had me slide almost off the table, spread my legs, and put my bare feet on the cold metal stirrups. I hardly saw the doctor, for as soon as he came in he sat on a stool between my legs, and the sheet hiked up by my knees was like a tent he was crawling into. What in the world was he doing in there? I felt odd sensations of discomfort, but the feelings were hard to locate, identify. It was embarrassing to have the nurse stand there while the doctor kept saying in a petulant voice, relax, relax. He meant muscles, not feelings.

After the exam I told him what I had told Dr. Schur.

"Do your mother and father know about this!" he exploded. "Did they bring you up to act this way? Did they? Did they?"

I couldn't speak. Tears clotted my throat, but he wouldn't make me cry, he wouldn't, wouldn't.

"I have three girls myself and I pray to God that when they get to be your age, they have the sense to save themselves for marriage. What have you got to look forward to now? And think how disappointed your husband will be! Think how *he'll* feel."

Angrily he scribbled out a prescription. "I guess I have to give you this. It's not against the law. There's no use getting pregnant on top of all this. But I'm not in the business of giving out contraceptives, so don't go telling all your little friends they can come here to get them." And with that, he swept from the room.

I had to use the sheet to wipe a big wet tear off my cheek.

I drove over to Joel's apartment that evening and found him in his gym shorts cooking spaghetti. He was so familiar and foreign to me. I sat at the table and burst into tears. When I was able to see again, there was his leg resting on the rung of the chair, and I remembered the first time I had met him.

"So tell me," he said nasally, in his accent.

"The doctor fussed at me. He said what would my parents say. He had no right to do that! No right to talk to me that way!"

"Good!" Joel said. "Good! That's the first time I've heard you mention your rights. Did you tell him to shove it?"

I looked at him, shocked. "What do you mean? I could never do a thing like that! I couldn't even speak! It's for you I'm doing all this!"

He sat down, grinning at me with his big white teeth. He was the only person I knew who brushed his teeth in the shower. "Oh, it's for me, is it? It is, huh? I didn't realize it was such a sacrifice." And he reached over and touched my breast. He was always doing unexpected, Northern things.

"I'm not like you," I said. "You can tell anybody off. Words come easy to you. I know you're older and smarter than me. Just don't tease me."

"Not smarter," he said. "Just older. Older, dear

Paulette, because there was never anyone as young as you." Then he stood and took me in his arms, as if he really did love me.

I wrote a letter to the editor of the *Daily Tarheel*, saying why coeds should be given birth control pills. The letter was full of yes's and no's and the word "meaningful." "Birth control pills are essential for the New Woman because they make her 'no' a meaningful one. The pill enables her to say 'yes' if she likes, and therefore if she chooses to say 'no,' that answer is a meaningful one. A 'no' has no meaning unless a 'yes' is possible."

I waited in fear and trembling for the letter to come out, in public. Then everyone would *know*. When it did, the headline said, "Pill Opens the Door."

Joel laughed when he read that. "That's not exactly what I meant," I said.

"It's all righteously ethical and philosophical," Joel said. "But why didn't you just say girls have the right to screw like everyone else, and the university is wrong to dictate morals?"

"But I did!"

I had lost my virginity, I had changed my life, but I had to admit that sex was a disappointment. The first thrill of going all the way (where?) had worn off, and now I felt like a bystander, watching someone else get something, but what? Joel seemed to get exactly what he wanted out of it, but in my own body I felt inarticulate, dumb. I didn't even have the first idea what my body would say if it could speak, in its own language. (I was twenty-one years old, and I didn't know that women had orgasms. Did other girls like me know about orgasms? This is the sort of question that needs to be asked at high school reunions.)

I couldn't get used to sleeping with Joel and his snoring, and I was homesick for my own bed. I was spending nearly every night with Joel, in his bed, and when I returned to my own apartment it had the appearance of a life suspended. One night I dreamed that two people I had known in high school were getting married. Everyone from school was there for the wedding. The couple had eyes that were just alike, huge and bronze. Everyone could see that they belonged together. As the wedding festivities were going on, in the dream I felt an unutterable sadness, and when I awoke the next morning, the feeling lingered on.

I started the pill, and at the end of the month, when it was time for my period, it didn't come. Being the New Woman was getting to be a strain. Joel was organizing a strike of underpaid black employees at the local cafeteria, and I was seeing less and less of him. The previous spring Martin Luther King had been assassinated. When I had heard of King's death, I came bursting into my dorm room. My roommate was lying in bed reading a magazine. She was engaged to an airline pilot, and took courses called "Kiddie Art" and "Kiddie Lit." Yes, she had heard. But what did you expect? she said to me. It was bound to happen sooner or later. I don't see why you're so upset. And she had gone back to reading her magazine.

Now I went here and there, too restless to sit still. I felt I had a slight fever all the time. My mind was electrified, I had a hard time making my body keep up with it. To make myself a little independent from my parents, I took a part-time job handing out towels at the gym. It didn't seem right to take their money when they would have died if they knew what I was doing. I avoided thinking about that as much as possible. I have to lead my own life, I would say to Joel, as if that were in doubt.

When I told him about missing my period, he insisted on a pregnancy test. On the way to the hospital, my sample bottle of urine in hand, I felt I had come to the worst day of my life. Anybody having a pregnancy test should be happily married with an extra bedroom. The test came out negative, and when I spoke to Dr. Schur, he said the pill had probably affected my cycle and to wait another month. Although I knew better, I felt I had gotten what I deserved.

At the end of the summer, I went home for my older sister's wedding. The wedding was like a Cecil B. DeMille movie. It was as if for her whole life, my mother had been preparing for this masterpiece of detail no one else actually cared about.

All the food, clothes, parties, and people made me sleepy and tense. I kept to myself as much as possible. My back ached the whole time, and I feared I had injured it somehow, lying unmarried under Joel Goldetski.

When I returned to campus in the fall, Joel did not get in touch with me, and though I was shocked, I had expected it. I felt very tragic for a few weeks, abandoned and all, but after a while I slept with another boy and then another, feeling very cavalier and complicated. Sometimes I would see Joel and the big white dog moving across campus in the old way. I would look away then, for there was something in the dog, the way he ran searching so, that reminded me of myself. Once there was a picture of Joel in the campus newspaper. He had been hit over the head with a bottle at a campus demonstration against the Vietnam War. For a while I tried to rouse the proper emotions regarding him—outrage, anger, hurt—but these were hard to sustain. After a while I wasn't sure who had left whom, or why. It was just that the summer had come to an end.

I moved into a one-bedroom apartment in an old house and worked long weekends at a little table near a window overlooking the yard. I was writing stories, and it took a lot of my time. Everything around me moved, and I moved, people came and went, I ran searching and didn't know what I wanted to find. In the spring I fell in love with a junior English major who wanted to be a lawyer, and I thought, this is it, finally, this is love, and it will last forever. But then I received a fellowship in writing to a university all the way across the country, and in spite of love, I knew I would be moving on, perhaps for a long time to come.

3

In May I turned thirty-nine, and my biological clock turned too, into a time bomb. But we were still in that no-man's-land (or no-child's-land) of *not-trying*. I knew one way to defuse the bomb would be to start *trying*—commencing all the icky things that people move on to when doing what comes naturally turns up empty: taking my temperature, charting my ovulation, timing intercourse, getting outside help if need be. But I couldn't do it.

I had been going along so nicely, I thought, my ducks if not in a row at least in a circle, thinking I knew who I was, that I understood my life, when suddenly I felt like one of those contestants on *To Tell the Truth*: Will the real me please stand up? Several of us did. There was the me who felt her heart would break if I didn't have a child, the me who felt her life would be over if I did, and the me who was stumbling around as if shell-shocked going "But . . . but . . . but . . ."

Then, right in the midst of all our *not-trying* that summer, my uncle H. C. died of cardiac arrest at the age of seventy-eight. I had always looked on my father, my uncle H. C., and my uncle Perry as an invincible triumvirate. Brothers, variations on the same theme, they grew up in the country, in a big white house in Marietta, South Carolina. As young men they all moved to Greenville, where I grew up, thirty miles away. They all spoke with that soft Southern accent particular to the upper Piedmont of South Carolina. All three of them were very gentle, very kind, very sweet. I had always assumed that the past, like the future, would always be there, but lately I was getting the feeling that I was wrong on both counts. Both were in danger of disappearing.

I didn't make it home for my uncle's funeral in July, and when I finally did get home to South Carolina in August, it was raining. Raining, after the worst drought in the Southeast's recorded history. All summer long, in Minnesota, I had watched the news reports on the South's hot dry summer, its suffering: hay lifts from the Midwest, farmers selling off cattle that were starving, lives ruined, people without air conditioning dying in their homes, their body temperatures over 100. I had suffered too, watching those reports. I dreamed of seeing my beloved South parched and brown, the kudzoo, dogwood, and azaleas done in, as if some terrible biblical plague had punished the South for its unfathomable sins. But it was raining. And coming into the airport in Greenville, from the air I saw what I saw every time I came home: green. Green fields and forests, materializing into pines as we banked to the left and came in on the one runway.

Jeff had not come with me for this trip. He made it to South Carolina about every other time, and I didn't mind. In fact, I enjoyed the chance to have my parents all to myself. My attention was always torn between him and them when I was home, and it wasn't easy to entertain him in Greenville. In a way it was a luxury to return to the past alone. It required my full concentration.

At the bottom of the airplane steps, an Eastern attendant was handing each passenger a big red-and-white umbrella. I walked toward the terminal in the rain, and there they were, crowding against the concrete railing at Gate Number 1: my mother, my father, looking miniature to me, old age having shrunk them from the larger-than-life figures of my childhood. I turned their ages over and over in my mind, trying to come to terms with them, trying to figure out the meaning. *Was it death?* Surely that was the message those numbers held, but one my mind rejected, firmly. I knew they would die, but I could not believe it. This paradox brought tears to my eyes, and perhaps to theirs—for my father was teary, my mother clingy—when I reached the big open space of white concrete that is the place of arrivals and departures in my life.

How funny my father looked! I laughed, a mixture of embarrassment and joy. He was wearing red-and-black polyester slacks, Hager perhaps, the very thing that a comedian had mocked in a show Jeff and I had gone to on Saturday night. I lived in two worlds, one where people laughed at such slacks, the other where my father wore them. I complimented him, for how could they be ignored, and he was proud of them, proud of himself. There was something childlike and innocent about him now that he was in his eighties. He could not speak at my arrival, choked as he was with emotion.

My mother was a more complicated case. Her mother-eyes took in everything—my clothes, my face, my posture, my purse, my shoes (were the heels run down?). I was being assessed, evaluated, to see how I was doing, in more ways than one. How complex and difficult my mother was, how ignorant and wise, kind and mean, helpful and hostile, powerful and weak, loving and afraid—any daughter's dream of a mother! How dependent I had felt on her, how much I had tried to protect myself from her, how I had needed and fled her.

"Are you feeling okay, honey?" my father asked solicitously as we walked to the car, a huge ancient gold Plymouth station wagon with wings.

"Are you hungry?" my mother asked when we got to the house. "I fixed a big pot of vegetable soup. Okra and fresh corn sheared off the cob and tomatoes I canned myself."

"There's corn muffins," my father said, "and some of that seven-layer salad Mother makes so good."

After I had eaten my fill, we sat in the den with the TV on. I told my parents that I wanted to research the family tree while I was home.

"Too bad H. C. isn't here to help you out," my father said. "He was real interested in the old folks."

Once Uncle H. C. sent me a letter someone had sent him about a big Bates clan that had lived around Marietta in the 1800s. The letter, from one sister to another, documented a husband and wife who had had twenty-one living children, and three dead ones. The woman, Sarah Springfield Bates, had married at fourteen and had her last living child at forty-five. She gave birth to another child, dead, at age fifty-one, and one of her dead children, the letter said, had been born with teeth in its mouth. When she died, her husband remarried and had seven more children.

That woman had had twenty-one children and I was worried about having one. How did she keep track of them all? Did she want so many children? Did she have other things she wanted to do with her time? But of course such questions were probably not in her mind. She probably hadn't had a lot of time for self-doubt.

The morning after I got in, I rushed down to the county courthouse to look into old wills. I was after a couple of my great-great-grandparents. My uncertainties about the future created a sudden need to fill in the past. Maybe by filling in names and dates on a sheet of paper, I could control whatever it was I felt streaming from me.

I hardly knew where to start. Going backward in time, things branched out, expanded exponentially. I needed days, weeks, months to do this work, slowly and thoroughly, but I felt like a chicken with its head cut off, running around hysterically. I raced up to deeds and over to the South Carolina room at the county library, photocopying things and ruining my eyes on ancient microfilm. That night when I got in, my parents were watching *Wheel of Fortune*.

"That Vanna," my father said proudly. "She's a local girl."

"North Myrtle Beach," my mother explained.

I showed my parents the documents I had copied. "Isn't it incredible!" I exclaimed. "They all lived around Marietta! They all came from the same small village!"

My parents looked at me as if they didn't know exactly what I meant.

"What are you going to do with all this . . ." my mother indicated my papers and ancestor charts, "when you get it all written down?"

Now it was my turn to look at her as if I didn't understand.

My mother had a ladies' luncheon for me while I was home. She invited my two childhood friends, Shirley and Cass, and their mothers, Mrs. Wainwright and Mrs. Blake.

Over the years I had lived away, these ladies' luncheons had become an institution. Whenever I came to town, my mother or one of the other mothers would get us all together. For the first few years after I left home, such get-togethers were something of an ordeal for me. I was living in California then, and I certainly wasn't doing things the way we had been brought up to do them. Shirley and Cass had stayed in town, married local boys, had children. There was always something I needed to keep quiet about: a lover, or, for four years there, the fact that I was living, unmarried, with Jeff. It didn't matter that my parents knew; social appearances had to be maintained. I was always afraid that over a glass of sherry or a piece of pecan pie I would lose my mind, crack under the pressure, and blurt out that I was living in sin. I didn't know whether my friends would have cared, but that was hardly the point. We had to keep up the front that we were nice Southern ladies, leading pure straight lives of moral correctness. I found it quite a strain.

Ladies' luncheons were also, for a period there, part of the complicated power struggle between my mother and me. She knew I'd just as soon avoid them, so she'd issue or accept an invitation before I got home, and there would be no way to back out. If I argued with her about it, she'd say she didn't see why I had to make such a fuss about seeing old friends. But I knew the agenda was more complicated than that. She wanted, I thought, to show me via Cass and Shirley how things should be, how daughters should live, and also, for my mother was never a simple case, she wanted to show me off, because she was proud of my accomplishments, despite my errant ways. Most of all, perhaps, she didn't want me to lose touch with my old friends, even if I sometimes did.

Over the years, however, I grew to see that at least in part my mother was right. As I became more comfortable with myself and more surely established in my own life, it became easier to accept my friends and the choices they had made. I wasn't so defensive or threatened. I found I enjoyed hearing about their lives in Greenville, and I was grateful for the continuity of those friendships, the love and loyalty we actually shared. I was glad my mother hadn't let me throw so much away.

So I was looking forward this visit to the very thing that I had once resisted. We would play our parts of Southern ladies of a certain race and class, full of warmth, charm, and a kind of self-deprecating humor which I enjoyed, but that didn't mean ladies' luncheons were my life (nor my friends'). Shirley and Cass would pass around pictures of their children, and Mrs. Blake and Mrs. Wainwright would fulfill their roles as doting grandmas, and then my mother would serve a lovely luncheon on Wedgwood china with the good silverware. We were having her chicken salad made with celery and pecans, along with a tomato aspic with olives set in a shimmering mold, and hot crescent rolls with butter. When did I ever get food like that? We'd top it off with the Milky Way chocolate cake that she and I had made the night before, happy as we stirred and baked.

Eventually, around three in the afternoon (we'd be exhausted!), the ladies would leave, and my mother and I would change out of our good clothes (these were the sweet moments) and relax in the kitchen by doing the dishes and putting up the food, letting our hair down and talking over what had occurred. We could be our real selves, not the ladies of a ladies' luncheon. I'd eat some leftover chicken salad, my favorite moment of the day, and then if we were lucky, we'd take a little nap.

And up to a point, that's the way it went. I was happy to see my old friends—Shirley, whom I had followed around in her horse pasture when she'd whistle for the horses like a man, and Cass, whom I had known since kindergarten, when we were both kittens in "The Three Little Kittens Who Lost their Mittens." (Oh! the gray-and-white felt kitten costume my mother made, with the long stuffed tail that I loved.) I hugged their thin backs, and embraced their mothers, those other mothers to me. How could I not be happy to see them all? I knew they had always loved me.

Almost as soon as we sat down, Shirley and Cass got out pictures of their children, and Mrs. Blake told how she had had to stay up until two in the morning to finish the formal she was sewing for her granddaughter's prom, and Mrs. Wainwright told us all about the school musical her grandson was in. My mother and I asked interested, animated questions in our roles of Southern hostesses, and after a while, we all trooped into the dining room and ate the chicken salad, which was great.

But then, after they had left, when my mother

and I were in the kitchen, doing the dishes, I said something to the effect of, "It seems all Shirley and Cass can talk about is their kids." There *had* been a good deal of conversation about offspring, and I was feeling a little insecure, sensitive, jealous perhaps. I was hoping my mother would agree with me, and then I'd feel supported in my life, which did not revolve around children.

My mother paused a moment in her dish washing, and then without looking at me, said, "Well, I'll tell you what I think. I think people who don't have children are the most selfish people in the world."

Hot and cold passed over me. My face stung, as if I'd been slapped. Something was being communicated here. It was directed at me. But even as I reeled inside, I knew that I had to stand up to her. "Mother," I said tightly, "do you mean me?"

She paused again, perhaps testing how far she dared go. "No," she said. Then after a moment she added, "Not yet."

"How can you say such a thing!" I said. "I know people who have children who are plenty selfish, and . . ."

But the moment had passed. It wasn't worth arguing about. I had been attacked and, in spite of my defenses, hit. We finished the dishes mostly in silence, and I consoled myself that in a few days, I could escape to Minneapolis. I would tell my women friends, *You'll never guess what my mother said to me while I was home!* But in the meantime, I had to get through our visit. I loved my mother. I loved her every bit as much as, at a moment like this, I hated her.

After we finished the dishes, I told my mother I wanted to visit the zoo. It was as good an excuse as any to get away. Where my mother was concerned, I was always escaping and always returning.

I walked down McDaniel toward Cleveland Park. The sidewalk here was buckled and broken from the roots of ancient pin oak trees. I crunched acorns as I went, stepping over the silvery trails of slugs. Minneapolis would never tolerate such sidewalks as these. They'd be out with jackhammers and cement mixers, making the way smooth for pedestrians, charging the homeowners. I rested my eyes in the deep shade of someone's yard: azalea bushes, a huge magnolia, dogwoods. Whenever I passed into a patch of sunlight, the heat pressed me like a hot hand.

"People who don't have children are the most selfish people in the world." I had never heard such a compressed bit of speech in my life.

I hadn't realized my mother was so angry with me. But seeing my friends must have reminded her of how I had let her down. I hadn't done the female thing, I hadn't had a child.

She obviously wanted to punish me in the worst way she knew how: by calling me selfish. *The most selfish person in the world.*

Well, that did go right to the heart of things. I

was selfish. Self-ish. Self-ish had been my goal since leaving home. To have a self. To be a self.

Had my mother felt, in having us, that she had had to give up her own "selfish" desires? Was she saying, in effect, that she had sacrificed in having us, and now she was mad—MAD—that I was getting off the hook? I was going blithely about my life, doing exactly what I wanted, ignoring my female destiny, and it was an outrage. An *outrage!*

I thought there was an element of that.

But I also knew my mother hadn't regretted having my sister and me. She loved us—that much was clear. She would say, if I asked her, that having us had been worth every bit of it, whatever "it" entailed. It occurred to me that she was angry at me at least in part because I was about to miss out on what she considered the most important thing in the world. Her words were an attempt, albeit a crude one, to bully me into motherhood, for my own good.

My mother and father waited a long time to have children. They said they wanted to be financially stable before they started a family. But I liked to think maybe they were having fun—young, married, living in Greenville away from their old-fashioned, Southern Baptist country parents. They had met in Marietta on one of the trips back to South Carolina that my mother's parents made from Texas, where they had moved shortly after they were married. My mother was sixteen, my father twenty-six. His first sight of her was her legs; he was lying under his car, tightening something up. He said he'd wait for her to grow up, and in the meantime, he drove to Texarkana to see her in his shiny black Model A Ford.

She had two years of community college in Texarkana, and then my father arranged for a teaching job for her in Marietta; his father was chairman of the school board. She roomed with relatives while my father courted her, though she has said that she wasn't in love with him at first, he was such an "old man." She just liked to ride in his car. At twenty she married the old man, and taught school and piano while my father got established in the electronics business. Finally, after twelve years of marriage, they had my sister in 1944, and three years later they had me. My mother was thirty-five when I was born, my father forty-five. Did someone say to my mother during those childless years that it was selfish not to have children? My mother had liked teaching, she liked making the money. But she stopped teaching after Betty was born, and she never worked outside the home after that. She was ready, she said, to devote herself mind and body to us from then on, which might be one reason why I was having so much trouble deciding about children myself.

I walked quickly along the jogging path in Cleveland Park. No one was about, and here along the banks of the muddy Reedy River, it was quiet, cool. Across the way I could see the old red skating rink building where we came to skating parties as children; the refreshments were always Krispy Kreme donuts and cartons of ice cold Pet milk. Farther on was the former site of the park swimming pool, which the city had shut down in the early sixties on account of integration. They filled it with dirt and planted roses, rather than let black children swim.

I came to the dark granite Vietnam Memorial. I always stopped here when I came to the park. I was drawn to the inscription engraved on the stone:

> *The young warrior does not speak.*

> *Nevertheless, he is heard in the still houses:*
> *Who has not heard him.*
> *He has a silence that speaks for him at night*
> *and when the clock counts.*

> *I am young. I have died. Remember me.*

Fourteen thousand young men and women from Greenville served during the Vietnam War, I read through blurry eyes. Now we knew that many of them had been poor, many black. I looked at the names of the dead carved in stone. One hundred and four of them. You would think that after so many years, the grief would be done. But here it was again, right in my chest.

I walked on, more slowly now. I had only known one boy killed in Vietnam—Andy Miller, who used to cannonball off the diving platform at Table Rock

State Park lake, where we had a summer cabin. He had lapis blue eyes, black straight hair that fell into his face, and a belly that jiggled with baby fat above his red plaid Janzen bathing suit. He was always jumping off the high dive, balling himself into a bomb to splash the bedickens out of the other kids around the tower, fifteen years old he was then, from a country family up there above Table Rock, and me wondering idly on my towel on the beach if he'd make a good boyfriend, a good husband, as I wondered about every boy back then. What about his choices? From the grave, my tortuous debate over procreation would seem a sad joke to him; an incredible luxury.

The zoo was built on terraces on a red dirt hill covered with trees and shrubs. As I neared I heard strange jungle noises, howls, hoots, screams. I paid my three dollars at the gate, and pushed through the turnstile. Before I reached it I smelled a stench coming from the elephant exhibit. Here was Joy II, Joy I having been the elephant of my childhood before this zoo was built. Joy II stood on a rock surface, separated from us by a moat, swinging a tire with her strange trunk. Her big gray ears were fanning back and forth. She had been donated, I read, by Burger King and WFBC-TV. Some new viewers arrived, a mother and two children, who laughed spontaneously at the sight of Joy. "Hey, Joy-ee!" the little girl called out in her Greenville twang. (Did I ever sound like that, before I moved away and got so sophisticated?) "How can she do that?" the little boy asked of the tire swinging. "She's wonderful."

At that moment Joy turned her big back end to us and farted. The fart bellowed out the folds of skin around her rectum with its windy force. I laughed, and thought to myself, "How can she do that?" Obviously Joy-ee was full of tricks.

I wandered on, pausing at the white-cheeked gibbons who sat high on tree branches at the top of their cages, frowning down at the human parade. Next door were colobus monkeys from Mount Kenya, with their huge plumey white tails and long black fur coats trimmed in white, the most elegant of costumes. Where animals were concerned, God certainly had a good imagination.

After the black-and-white ruffed lemurs, the red ruffed lemurs, and the ring-tailed lemurs, I was lemured out. I sat down on a bench in the shade.

Across the way a female peacock—peahen?— walked almost camouflaged among the brown pine needles, two chicks sheltering under the broad umbrella of her body, moving when she moved, stopping when she stopped. They seemed like little brown pieces of herself pinched off. She had her head up and moved cautiously, anxiously scanning for danger, the classic mother pose. Something about it made me flinch. And where was the peacock? I spotted him down the hill, bumming popcorn from strangers.

A memory came back to me, from a long time

ago. I must have been just a toddler, maybe two years old. We were at Myrtle Beach, and I had been left on the blanket while my parents and sister were down at the ocean's edge, playing in the surf. Suddenly a monster with weird eyes on sticks (a sand crab, I later learned) rose out of a hole in the sand. Those eyes on sticks looked right at me. I screamed bloody murder, and my mother came running, swooping me up against her wet black bathing suit, asking me what was wrong. How could I tell her? I could only blubber and point to a hole in the sand, but I remember the comfort in rejoining her wet mother-body.

I thought of the summer between first and second grade, when she worked with me at the big pine table on the screened porch at our cabin at Table Rock. I had a lisp. I couldn't pronounce "s's." I had discovered this one day while standing with my feet in the chain link fence that separated our yard from that of the Willises. All the neighborhood kids had gathered around and were asking me how old I was. Tix, I told them proudly, thrilled to be the center of attention. How old? they asked again, as if they were deaf. What was so funny? I told them again and they asked me again, over and over, until finally I stamped my foot on the ground and burst into tears. All that summer my mother worked with me, the speech therapy books spread out before us, while my sister and Jimmy and Johnny, our cousins from the cabin next door, ran outside to play. She put my tongue through the tongue twisters over and over, the way a circus trainer puts his ponies through hoops. By the start of second grade I could say "start," "second," and "say."

But then I thought of how she made lists for us of chores to do, and how we had to make our bed every single morning, even on Christmas! She was always after us to practice the piano, calling out B-flat! or A-sharp! from the kitchen when we hit a wrong note. We had to have clean white gloves on Sunday morning, and write thank-you notes for every gift. She couldn't look at Betty and me without thinking up some way to improve us, something else that we needed to do. No wonder we wanted to escape her.

So much was involved in being a mother! Too much.

Another memory surfaced, from a long time ago. It was Mother's Day, and we had come home from church in our Sunday clothes, with roses—red for my mother, sister, and me because our mothers were still living, and white for my father because his mother was dead—pinned on our lapels. Our father gave our mother a Mother's Day gift, a big new frying pan, perhaps one of the first electric ones. My mother opened the big beautifully wrapped package happily, but when she saw what it was, she let it crash to the floor. "I don't want anything else to cook with or have to clean up!" she shouted and ran from the room, slamming the door to their bedroom with a resounding bang. My father, sister, and I stared at each other in shock. We were frightened and confused. We had never seen our mother react in such a way. Didn't she like being a wife and mother? Didn't she like to cook and clean up? We had assumed that was *who she was*. But here was some new information. If she didn't want a new frying pan, if she didn't want to always be taking care of us, what did she want? Even at age eleven that question caused my heart to flip, my stomach to drop.

What was it she had wanted? She had everything she was *supposed* to have. And yet there was something . . . I didn't even know what it was, but I must have felt what was missing, for I had continued the search myself.

She had wanted me to be in the talent show when I was in seventh grade. She had studied "Recitation" in school and produced an ancient text of monologues from which she chose one for me: "Fauntleroy's Wail." We spent hours drilling, with her coaching me on which words to emphasize, which gestures to make. For the show I wore black knickers, a white ruffled shirt, and a red cummerbund. I was Bobby, a country bumpkin dressed as Little Lord Fauntleroy by his mother who had read a book about him by "Frances Hogeater Burman." My first lines were, "There ain't no pleasure in being a boy these days, there ain't! I'd almost as soon be a girl." Given my tender gender identity at thirteen, no wonder I got mixed up.

It wasn't a great success. Although I tried to sound perky and ham it up the way we had practiced, I performed in a stilted paralysis of fear, embarrassment, and self-consciousness. But even as I hated the whole business, I understood what my mother was after, though nothing was ever said. She wanted me to have experiences, opportunities, find a talent if I had one. I sensed that she came down on the side of Bobby's mother, who might be accused of putting on airs, but at least she had a vision.

It was around this time that I discovered writing. I had as my speech teacher that year an unmarried woman (old maid, as we thought back then) named Miss Harvard, who had a passion for literature. She'd stand on her desk with her chiffon scarves wrapped around her neck (am I making this up?) and recite Vachel Lindsay's "The Congo": *Boom-a-lay, boom-a-lay, boom-a-lay, boom!* She had us write a short story, something I had never done before.

There was nothing in my background that would indicate I'd take to writing. My parents were not readers, really. My father would thumb through the yellow *National Geographic*s that came to the house in brown paper wrappers (and I would too, looking for pictures of women's breasts, which was probably what he was looking for—the closest I came back then to sex education). But my mother had some books left over from her younger days: Gene Stratton Porter's *A Girl of the Limberlost* and *The Keeper of the Bees*, which I devoured, wondering if Gene was a woman, not realizing there was another spelling of the name for a female.

And Mother had an old book from college, *Selec-*

tions from American Literature, which I pored over
constantly: Whitman, Hawthorne, Longfellow, Poe,
Twain, O. Henry. There was one poem in the book,
by Joaquin Miller (I didn't know how to pronounce
Joaquin), titled "Kit Carson's Ride," which I read
hundreds of times. No matter how often I read it, it
never failed to move me. A dramatic monologue, it
tells how Kit Carson and his stolen Indian bride
have to outrun a prairie fire on horseback. Carson's
horse, Pache, is blinded by the fire as he carries the
two of them to the safety of the Brazos River. I
couldn't get enough of this poem: its drama, its im-
ages, its rhythm, its emotion. "Aye ride for your lives,
for your lives you must ride! For the plain is aflame,
the prairie's on fire . . ." The ending never failed to
bring tears to my eyes:

> *I look'd to my left then—and nose, neck, and shoulder*
> *Sank slowly, sank surely, till back to my thighs,*
> *And up through the black blowing veil of her hair*
> *Did beam full in mine her two marvelous eyes,*
> *With a longing and love yet a look of despair*
> *And of pity for me, as she felt the smoke fold her,*
> *And flames leaping far for her glorious hair.*
> *Her sinking horse falter'd, plunged, fell and was gone*
> *As I reach'd through the flame and I bore her still on.*
> *On! into the Brazos, she, Pache and I—*
> *Poor, burnt, blinded Pache. I love him . . . that's why.*

So I was ready when Miss Havard asked us
seventh-graders to write a short story. I didn't know

I was ready, but I was. It was all there waiting for me, the desire and even the ability, imbibed no doubt from reading. The story unfolded in front of me like a big wave I could ride all the way in to shore. During the writing, I forgot for a little while that I was in junior high, quite a relief. And there the thing was, in black and white, nailed down on the page, where I could read it over and over when I had finished, and get the same feeling every time.

Oddly, the story had a middle-aged male narrator who looks up an old war buddy who once had the reputation of a wild playboy, the kind who loves 'em and leaves 'em. Only now the man is married and has seven (count 'em) children, and the thing is, his wife is no beauty. But she has *inner* beauty. Inner beauty was becoming very important to me in the seventh grade. I was playing out some fantasy in which the good girl wins out in the end. No wonder I got hooked on writing.

Miss Harvard picked my story out of the pile and read it to the class. I listened, enthralled. It really was a story, with a beginning, middle, and end. It was such a good story (I thought) that I almost forgot I had written it. Miss Harvard announced that I had talent. She invited my mother and me to tea (I had never been in an *apartment*), and it was there, under the tutelage of my mother and Miss Harvard, who had discovered their mutual interest in recitation and in my budding writing talent, that I first formulated the idea that I would be a writer.

Years later, when I wanted to transfer to the University of North Carolina so that I could take writing courses, it was my mother I petitioned. It wasn't that my father wasn't encouraging, it was just that Mother was the Minister of Education and Culture, the one who would understand. And by my senior year, when the writing fellowship came, I was ready to make the big leap, the leap that would take me all the way across the country, all the way away. And while it was true that I wanted to escape her, it was also true that whatever it was in me that was able to make that leap had come from her.

When I get in, my mother is standing at the stove heating streak o' lean in oil so that she can fry some okra. I suddenly realize how hungry I am and that dinner will be good.

"How was the zoo?" she asks me as if nothing has happened between us, and I tell her, as if nothing has happened between us, about the animals I've seen. "You would have enjoyed it," I say. "Joy II farted and about blew these two little kids away."

My mother laughs and I laugh, too. I want to be still mad at her, but in her presence anger is hard to maintain. She is too familiar to me, too important. I stand there watching her roll the cut okra in the cornmeal mix in an aluminum bowl with her bare hands. She lifts the fried fatback out with a fork and drains it on paper towel on a plate. When it is cool enough, I break off little bits of it with my fingers and melt that warm, salty fat in my mouth. I never fry okra myself, never buy fatback, but all my life I have stood by the stove while my mother fried okra.

"Mother," I say suddenly, surprising myself with my misery, "do you think Jeff and I should try to have a child?"

My mother without missing a beat: "You'd make a wonderful mother! I can't imagine you going through life without having children."

"But I don't know the first thing about babies! I wouldn't know what to do with one. You'd have to help me."

My mother: "I'll start reading up on it."

4

As I continued to try not only to recollect my life, but to make sense of it, certain moments stood out, certain turning points, as it were, the significance of which I had only dimly grasped at the time. It was scary, in retrospect, to see how fragile the circumstances surrounding these pivotal events seemed. Suppose, for example, that I had not had Miss Harvard for speech in seventh grade. I had had, let's say, Mr. Warren, who loathed reading student stories. Would I have missed, then, that small window of opportunity for discovering the fledging writer in myself? I suppose I would have come to it at another time by another route. But it seemed in some mysterious way that I had to have had Miss Harvard, that it could have only happened as it did.

Another of these pivotal events that seemed a strange mixture of both luck and fate involved a letter. One spring day my senior year I was sunning in the backyard of the old house where I rented my apartment in Chapel Hill. I was like the lily of the field, I sowed not nor did I reap, and I had no idea what I would do when I graduated in June. I had never gotten around to taking any education courses; I'd been too busy taking writing courses. I had applied to graduate school in writing because some of my teachers had encouraged me, for what I liked best was sitting at the round table in my dilapidated apartment, looking out the window, writing stories for class.

The postman came through the backyard, wearing blue shorts, with a handsome leather postal bag that I admired slung over his shoulder. He handed me a thin airmail letter that projected importance. My name was perfectly typed, on an IBM machine.

I had won a Wallace Stegner Fellowship in creative writing to Stanford University. The fellowship was named for a famous writer I had never heard of. In fact, I had barely heard of Stanford, and I kept confusing the name in my mind, sometimes calling it Sanford when I told people the places I'd applied to graduate school.

A week later I got a phone call from a man in New York. I had won a Book-of-the-Month Club Fellowship. Three thousand dollars.

I bought a car with the money. My father helped me pick it out, a Chevy Nova, perfect for a daughter like me.

I drove to California in the Nova with a boy I had picked up in Europe. My parents had given me the trip as a graduation present. They had been to Italy, Hawaii, and Japan themselves on trips my father had won as an RCA dealer. My girlfriend Darla and I visited my sister and her serviceman husband in Germany, and Darla's grandmother in Denmark. We had intended to visit museums in Italy, but we threw in the cultural towel and followed some Canadian boys to the Greek Isles. On the island of Ios I drank too much ouzo, ate something that made me sick, and passed out during the night when I got up to get a drink of water. The crack my head made hitting the stone floor of the room we were renting woke Darla up. When I came to, I figured I would die, but I didn't mind too much. I had been so happy on Ios, turning golden in the Mediterranean light, swimming every day in the blue-green sea. I didn't die, but I did get a big knot on my head and had to stay in bed a few days. Old Greek women in black came to visit me, bearing red carnations. They'd slowly open and close the door to remove the flies, making the room light and dark, light and dark.

It was hard to explain to my mother exactly what I had in mind driving across the country with a boy I had met in Europe. "Mama, just look at it this way. If I have car trouble, I won't be all alone way out in the middle of nowhere."

"You aren't going to sleep in the same motel room, are you?"

"Oh, no, it's nothing like that!"

Sex hung in the air, unspoken. My mother was fixing some pimiento cheese sandwiches, pound cake, and a thermos of coffee for the trip.

"You better not let your father know about this."

Actually, I didn't think my father would get it. He left my sister's and my repression up to my mother.

"And you don't even know him," my mother said, not looking at me. "Someone you picked up in Europe. A stranger."

Steve wasn't so strange at all. He was nice enough, if a little dull. He was enrolled at Chico State, and he was enamored of me mainly because he was enamored of Stanford. I was going to pick him up outside Atlanta, where he had been visiting his sister.

Out in the driveway my father was checking the Nova, making sure it had oil, gas, window spray. He and my mother had been so proud of me for winning the fellowship to Stanford and the Book-of-the-Month Club money. My picture had been in the paper. I was smiling graciously as if people won fellowships and money all the time.

"You better stop every hundred miles or so," my mother said uncertainly. "And let him do most of the driving." She paused for a long moment, as if making up her mind. "Maybe he doesn't even know what pimiento cheese is. I better fix a few ham and cheese."

In the end she'd rather have me protected than pure, and perhaps she knew I was already gone.

California was a big surprise to me. I had expected it to be so pastoral, a place where horses graze on hills, and I was not prepared for the Bayshore Freeway. I was glad Steve was driving. He put me up at his parents' house for a few days in Redwood City, and helped me find an apartment in Palo Alto, a one-room efficiency in the back of a big house on Cowper Street, one block off University Avenue. I decorated my tiny place with my collection of hats: bolero, beret, felt, straw, and floppy. In pictures from that time—1969—I am wearing very short skirts, my hair is long and straight, and my glasses are granny, tinted brown.

I knew California was the place to be. I had seen the television reports of Haight-Ashbury, with its children of peace and love. I might not be ready for the Haight, but I was only thirty miles away. Even more important, I was three thousand miles from home. I had managed to escape the South, with its big eye, always watching me, always judging me. I thought of California as a place of freedom, especially sexual freedom. I was very interested in sexual freedom. I remember standing in White Plaza that first year at Stanford listening to Germaine Greer talk in public about women's orgasms. She was a tall, beautiful, fierce woman, and though my face burned in embarrassment, my heart leapt at her words. I had not yet had an orgasm, and I was coming to the uncomfortable understanding that something had been taken from me, never given to me. I sensed that sex was connected to self. There were certain words in the air—sexuality, choice, independence, autonomy, self. They were new words to me, but once I heard them, I knew instinctively that they were the right words, the necessary words.

I was so happy to be at Stanford, which I now never mispronounced. It raised my IQ ten or fifteen points just to be there. I loved walking down Palm Drive to the campus with its Spanish mission architecture and red tile roofs. Behind the campus the foothills were a tawny yellow, with live oaks twisted into artistic shapes, and there, incredibly, a few horses did graze. It was only a forty-five-minute drive over the Santa Cruz Mountains to the Pacific Ocean. Sometimes big fog banks would roll in off the coast to hang on the lip of the foothills. The air and light were entirely different from that of the South; everything was different.

The advanced fiction-writing seminar met in the Jones Room in Building 50, where the English department was housed. Wallace Stegner, the famous writer for whom my fellowship was named, was our teacher. Was there ever a kinder, wiser face? He was a distinguished father figure who was about to win the Pulitzer Prize.

I was the youngest Stegner Fellow and, though I hadn't realized it before, something of a hick. I hadn't been a hick in Greenville. In Greenville I knew who the hicks were, and I hadn't been one of them. But at Stanford I was being exposed right and left to things I had never known about before. I remember going to a party thrown by a rich Jewish girl from New York. She asked me if I cared for Cointreau. I didn't know what it was. I thought it was some kind of cake. That was the kind of education I was getting at Stanford. It wasn't all books.

Stanford was actually giving me money to develop as a writer. But that was also a little frightening. Surely a lot was expected of me. What? Writing. They were giving me all this money (well, enough to live on for a year), so I figured they must expect big things from me. I was twenty-two years old, and the little writing I had done had come fairly easily to me, rather unself-consciously. Now, in the workshop, I was exposed to people who knew a lot more about literature and writing than I did. We sat around a big table, critiquing each other's stories. I felt young, Southern, and female. I was afraid I would say something dumb or wrong, while most of the others seemed able to spout off at will. It occurred to me that where writing was concerned, I didn't know what I was doing.

A few weeks after I arrived at Stanford I got a cat. I had always loved cats. I got my first cat when I was seven. I came home in my Brownie outfit, and my father was kneeling in the backyard, his hands in a cardboard box: inside were two black kittens. Tippytoes, because to me cats always seemed to be walking on their toes, and Tommy, because my mother said Tommy could be either a boy's name or a girl's name, and we didn't know which Tommy was, yet.

After Tippytoes and Tommy, who were, of course,

girls, a long line of cats. Cats and kittens, with their sure sense of self. They had always been there in my life, lazing in the driveway, prowling through my father's garden, mysterious and familiar, at home and yet apart, always there in my life, until they became a part of my life, a part of myself. Really, there was nothing I liked better.

Then for a few years there, while I was in college, I didn't have a cat. But now that I was on my own in California, I got one. Actually, it got me. One day a big black Persian with beautiful white markings on its face, chest, and feet addressed me on the street. It did not act particularly needy as if it were lost and abandoned. And yet it communicated to me that it was ready for a home: my home. It was such a beautiful cat that I tried, sincerely, to find its owner, for surely someone did love it. But no signs were posted in the neighborhood, no ads appeared in the Lost and Found, and when I called the pound, no one had reported such a cat as missing. I gave it every chance, out my back door, to go home, but it was home. That much seemed clear. It even had a name: Charlotte. I don't know how I knew the name. It was just that when I looked at the cat, who regarded me so calmly, so warmly, with round yellow eyes, I knew its name was Charlotte.

Having Charlotte, I felt more secure. Charlotte was such a mature, measured sort of personality, a great comfort to me in my own immaturity and uncertainty. It was as if I were free to engage in a few (for me) heartbreaking adventures as long as Charlotte held down the home front, a solid, accepting, unruffled presence for me to come home to. She was not nervous, and since I was, somewhat, most of the time, the sight of Charlotte, who had obviously arrived at some elevated philosophy about life, had a medicinal effect on my nerves.

I wanted to free myself sexually. I thought if I could be a sexually free woman, I would somehow be transformed into the intelligent, mature, sophisticated, independent individual I longed to be, but wasn't.

I was so sick of love. I had spent my whole life preoccupied with males: how to attract them; how to hold on to them. I didn't want to be a woman whose life revolved around a man; yet that was all I had ever known. I had breathed it in, it seemed, from everything around me: from books, from movies, from life itself. But now I was trying to learn something new—how to be the center of my own life. I had gone too far—all the way to California— to go back to the old ways, but they didn't die lightly. If only I could separate love and sex. Love was what tied women up; sex was what freed them.

There was the skinny hippie on a macrobiotic diet I met at the co-op. There was the lumberjack type I met on a walk in the woods, who pumped away and asked me every so often if I had come yet; there was the nice red-haired graduate student who was so sad over the breakup of his marriage that he couldn't get it up; and there was the journalism fellow who wanted me to use a vibrator on his butt, for all I knew a very California thing to do. There was this one and that one, and the more there were, the less free I felt, inside, where I was holding on very tight. I was not about to trust these strangers, no matter how much lip service I gave (and I gave a lot) to being free. Old scripts such as "take care of me forever" kept cropping up in my head.

One of the women I had gotten to know in the writing program told me how she was using a vibrator to satisfy her sexual needs, so she didn't have to depend on a man. She told me I could buy one in one of the porn shops along El Camino Real. Finally I screwed (so to speak) my courage up to go get one. Everything stopped when I came in the door. There were only men in there, that much I could tell, and I was, to say the least, an unusual customer. The man behind the counter was the kind of person whom my parents had always hoped to protect me from, but I tried to act nonchalant, as if young, virginal types such as I visited porn shops frequently to buy huge phallic-shaped vibrators. There they were, along with a number of other items, in a display case. My eyes blurred, instinctively protecting me from objects that I could hardly identify, and wouldn't know the use for. I didn't know whether I should ask to see a couple, as one might ask to see rings in a jewelry store, nor did I know what I would be appraising—the heft in my hand? The power? I wanted to make sure I didn't flinch, but on the other hand, why prolong the agony? I purchased a big beige one that seemed about a foot long, which I figured ought to do the job, and forced myself to walk out the door at a fairly normal pace. I took it home and quickly made friends with it.

Mr. Stegner was my adviser, and one day he asked me if I intended to go on for my master's degree. I was taking graduate courses in literature while on the fellowship, but I hadn't thought too much about actually getting the degree.

"I don't want to teach," I told him "I want to write"

He looked at me in his kindly way. I always got the feeling he knew things about which I didn't have a clue. "But you may need to make a living one day," he said, "and teaching is not such a bad way. The degree might come in handy."

He asked if I'd like to house-sit for him and Mrs. Stegner that summer while they were in Vermont. It would give me a free place to live, and then I could continue in the writing program and work on my master's in the fall.

I did house-sit for the Stegners that summer, and at the end of my first year in California, I traded in my Chevy Nova for a used Volkswagen camper. I didn't have a tape deck, but I did have a tape recorder so that when I drove around I could play the tape from Woodstock. I was not a hippie, but I was also not the daughter my parents had seen off in the little gray Nova. The camper was a compromise: a cross between the hippie vans I admired and was a little afraid of, the ones painted with rainbows and reeking of marijuana, and a small-scale Winnebago. I was counterculture in a middle-class way. I had a bed to sleep in, a miniature sink and icebox, and a top that popped up. When I traveled down the highway, my shadow resembled a loaf of bread.

When it was time for me to return to Stanford in September, I told my parents that I intended to drive to California by myself. I had had a rider to share driving and expenses on the trip home to South Carolina, but now I was determined to drive back alone. My poor parents. They were scared to death. They couldn't imagine their darling young daughter, whom they had always tried so hard to protect, doing such a thing. It was outside their experience, their imagination. It was also outside mine, which was the whole point. I was out to prove something to my parents, and even more important, to myself. The idea that I was a Southern young lady, by defi-nition someone who needed others to take care of her, had been built into me at a deep level. I figured if I could drive all the way across the country alone, I could probably do anything. I wouldn't have to depend on others; I wanted to depend on myself.

It was a long, uneventful trip. As I recall, I got

very sleepy every afternoon. Now I wonder why anyone would want to do such a thing—drive a Volkswagen camper three thousand miles alone. I see now that it's not that monumental. I'm not confusing myself with Amelia Earhart. It was only driving, after all. But at the time, for someone like me, it was a big thing.

I remember only one incident from the whole trip. One of the nights I was on the road, somewhere in the indeterminant middle, I checked into a motel just off the highway, as I did every night. I would eat dinner self-consciously in the motel restaurants, a very young-looking young woman with long straight hair, like Marianne Faithfull's. And because I was young, female, and alone, men would look at me. They would watch me. That was part of why I had to do it. I wanted to be able to withstand their stares, and still go on. I wanted to be able to move through the world on my own.

That night, when I had gone to my room—a generic motel room with a bed, a dresser, a window in front covered by a heavy curtain—there came a knock at the door. This was on a different order from my escapades at Stanford, where I was always pretty sure I was in control of the situation. I had the door locked, but I froze in place. I knew who it was. A man who had been watching me in the restaurant. Now he was knocking at my door. It had to do with sex. I was shocked and frightened. And all the more determined. He was knocking at my door simply because I was young, female, and alone. I hated him with all my heart. I knew he could stop me from moving through the world on my own.

That's all. He went away. I went to bed, shivering under the covers. And even though I was frightened to death, of everything, I did have a little nerve. Somewhere inside me I had a little nerve.

Charlotte and I moved into an airy apartment above a garage; it reminded me of being in a treehouse. I had survived my first year at Stanford, and now I was back for a second. I was full of hope and energy for the future. But I had also begun to understand that there was more to being a writer than simple desire. For one thing, I thought of Stanford as basically a male institution. It didn't strike me as a bit odd that I, a female student, was called a "Stegner Fellow." I assumed that writers *were* fellows. Men got to be writers, and women took care of them and their children. Of course I knew there were female writers—I was reading a number of them: Katherine Mansfield, Katherine Anne Porter, Virginia Woolf, Flannery O'Connor, Eudora Welty. But I didn't believe that they were women *and* writers. By women I meant wives and mothers. They seemed to be writers in spite of being women.

It made no real difference to me that an occasional female could slip by if she were exceptional and lucky, and had incredible talent and drive. I was pretty convinced that I didn't have incredible talent and drive. I had some talent and some drive. But deep down inside I believed that little girls grew up to be wives and mothers, and that little boys grew up to have work, and that work could be writing.

It was a time of consciousness-raising, and my consciousness needed raising. I joined a women's group. All the women in the group were at Stanford, either writers or doctoral students. The best and the brightest, you might say, or at least above average, and all scared in various ways, all remarkably similar in terms of self-doubt. We shared so many social, sexual, and academic insecurities that we had to believe that the problems lay not in us, but in society, the system, history, patriarchy, our families, our lovers. None of us thought about having children. We talked a lot about giving birth, but we meant to ourselves. Mainly, in spite of ourselves, we talked about our relationships with men. We didn't want to marry; but we would like to live with someone, and some of us did, off and on. We felt that our former selves—the girl-selves we had been back in our hometowns—were embarrassingly wrong, and we strove to reform. We said to each other that we must turn away from taking care of others and learn to take care of ourselves. We believed in making choices. Nothing in my background had encouraged me to think in terms of choices.

Stanford caught on and brought Tillie Olsen to campus to teach women's studies and fiction writing. I had never met a *woman writer*, and here one was, live and in person, taking my hand, squeezing it. I sat next to her at a campus movie, shyly, and was amazed when she put her feet up on the seat in front of us—so I did, too. When I read "Tell Me a Riddle" I wept, and understood that I was in the presence of greatness. Here was a story I would read over and over for the rest of my life, and it wasn't written by a man, someone dead or living in New York.

Tillie taught the graduate fiction seminar, so I signed up. I had grown more and more intimidated the previous year, especially by the men in the group. They seemed to have no internal blocks the way I did; they seemed confident, certain that what they wrote and said was important. They possessed a sense of entitlement that I simply didn't feel. All my life I had tried to be as feminine—as self-effacing, modest, humble, *nice*—as possible. These were not attributes for writing, it appeared. The men seemed to know more about work than I did: how to get the writing done; how to put the writing first; how to put themselves first.

One day one of the men in the seminar read a story that was written from a woman's point of view. It was about entering silence, and getting near the void. I should have been the one writing about silence, since I was finding it harder and harder to write. The story wasn't about the social and political factors that silence women. It was full of highly poetic, literary language, which certainly impressed me. Clearly the author had no trouble himself with silence.

Tillie lit right into it, saying it had nothing to do with a real woman. *With a woman's real life*, she said. She called it a complete romanticization of a woman's life, a man's theoretical usurpation of a woman's life! I was shocked, astounded. I had never thought about literature from a woman's perspective. And, of course, Tillie Olsen was the wrong one to mess with about women's silences. She was in the process of writing a book called *Silences*, which would become a classic of feminist literature.

I took Tillie's course in women's literature that year. We read *Daughter of Earth*, Sylvia Plath's poetry, *The Story of an African Farm*, *The Dollmaker*, *The Awakening*, and *To the Lighthouse*. My notebook was peppered with such phrases as "the accessibility of an open door. The privacy, the chance for concentration of a closed door . . ."; "silences of women who have never written . . ."; "born with a gift when the time is not such that you can use it . . ."; "In reading, what are the realities of women's lives? What is the difference in lives permitted men and women? What power did women have, and in what ways powerless?" "There is an awful 'yes' in every women's constitution (Dickinson)"; "Katherine Anne Porter on Hardy: 'His women are in the classic mold—they love, they suffer; his men are in the classic mold—they act, they try to change the circumstances of their lives'"; "after marriage, going about in a private totalitarian state"; "'Young girls are poems—they shouldn't write them'!"; "Angel in the house"; "having to be a fountain of sympathy and a mirror"; "What is it about Mrs. Ramsey that makes Lilly not want to marry?"

I showed Tillie one of my stories. I was worried that I wasn't any good, afraid that I didn't have anything to say. Tillie told me my story was clumsy and awkward. But still, she said, she cared for it more than anything she'd seen that quarter. You have the heart of a writer, she said.

I went out of her office with my heart in my hand. It quivered in ecstasy. I would work harder! I would write more! I knew my limitations—legion. I was not professional enough, I told myself harshly, firmly. I must work! I needed discipline, courage, determination. I was not particularly acquainted with discipline, courage, determination, but I recognized the value in them. I wanted them in my life.

Oh, Tillie! Your fierce eagle features, your dislocated speech, your neurotically tiny handwriting, your passion for the purity of art. You taught us well, and the lesson was, Don't be distracted. Don't get sidetracked. Don't let anything else consume you. Stay the course. Sit at your desk, and write.

This image then: a woman at a desk, writing. I see her in my mind: a woman at a desk, her head bent down, writing. Around her is great stillness and silence. There are only these things: the woman, the desk, writing. I want to be her. I want these things, and it seems in some ways that this is all I have ever wanted in my life: to be a serious person. To do serious work. It doesn't have to be important work, but it can't be bridge or knitting. It can be writing.

I have wanted to sit at my desk and work. Something that comes so easily for some people. But it is something that I have had to learn. Something I've had to work toward. Something I have failed at many times. To sit at a desk, writing. Something so plain and simple.

It has informed my life.

5

"Does anybody mind if I turn this on?" I put the tape recorder on the armrest between my father and his brother, my uncle Perry, in the front seat. We were on our way to the country, to Marietta, to look at graves.

My visit in Greenville was almost over. Tomorrow I'd be flying back to Minneapolis. I needed to get back to my life, back to Jeff, back to the future. I wondered what that future would hold.

Back at home Mother and Aunt Grace were finishing up the Sunday dinner dishes. They didn't share our interest in going to the country. They'd catch up with each other while we were gone, and have dessert ready when we returned.

I always saw Aunt Grace and Uncle Perry when I was home. They were like second parents to Betty and me, perhaps because they'd never had children of their own. Aunt Grace had had three miscarriages, and they didn't adopt. I had never thought much about their not having children when I was growing up, but now it had occurred to me that Jeff and I might turn out to be more like them than like our own parents.

There was a short silence while Uncle Perry adjusted to the idea of the tape recorder. Ostensibly it would save me taking a lot of notes, but I had an ulterior motive: I wanted to capture their voices on tape. Earlier that afternoon, after church, my father had helped me get it ready. He put in new "D" batteries and tested it in the den, saying, "Test, test, one-two-three-four testing," the way he used to test microphones for school assemblies and recitals.

"I don't know that I'll have anything to tell you," Uncle Perry said. He was eighty, tan from playing golf several times a week. In his Bermuda shorts, his legs were a deep golden brown, and the calf muscles were hard like those of a young man's, and hairless.

"Oh, I'm sure there'll be a lot," I said, opening my notebook.

"H. C. would have been the one to tell you," my father said. "He was real interested in the family." He pronounced "interested" in four distinct syllables.

In the backseat I was studying the lineage chart I had filled out. To the far right on the large sheet were lines for ancestors sixty-four through one-hundred and twenty-seven, none of which I had filled in. These flowed into boxes thirty-two through sixty-three, a few of which I had names for, and on down through my great-greats, my greats, and my grandparents finally to arrive at line number two, my father, and line number three, my mother. Then there was the space with my name filled in. I considered the blank that stemmed from Jeff and me.

It disturbed me to think of all those lives, my own included, coming to a halt with us.

"I don't know why I never got around to asking him," I said. "Let's see. Did you know your grandparents?"

My father and uncle were silent. I felt their memories working, searching, like slow computers.

"I don't know," my father said at last. "I can't remember."

"Both grandfathers were in the war," Uncle Perry said.

"Which war was that?"

"The War between the States. Both got wounded. In fact, I imagine that's what contributed to Grandfather Trammell's death. He got shot in the intestine and had to have an operation. Grandfather Bates walked with a cane."

My uncle pulled into the gravel driveway of the cemetery of Ebenezer Baptist Church. I remembered coming here as a child when my parents would put flowers on the graves. I had never asked much about these dead people back then. It was just an odd thing the grown-ups did, putting flowers on old graves.

We stood over my father's and Uncle Perry's parents' graves.

"We need a new load of gravel," my father said to Perry. "This one has about run away."

"Look how they're expanding across the road," Perry pointed out. "Looks like they're opening a whole new section over there."

I looked impatiently to where he was pointing. There was a split rail fence, and beyond, the new graves made me think of a housing project in the suburbs.

"What were they like?" I asked, nodding toward the graves.

My father rocked back on his heels, looking thoughtful. After a moment he said, "Perry'll have to tell you . . ."

Uncle Perry laughed softly. "Weren't you there?"

"When were they married?" I asked.

"I can't tell you when they were married," Uncle Perry said. "The Bates lived over on South Saluda River, and Dad married Elizabeth Trammel over on the North Saluda River. A good ways over there."

"The Trammells had a big piece of land over there," my father said. "Lots of good bottomland, and upland too."

"What was your mother like?" I asked. I was trying to balance my notebook on my tape recorder, an awkward arrangement.

"Dad was the rural mail carrier," my father said. "We used to ride all over these hills with him when he made his deliveries, first in a horse and buggy and then in a Model T Ford. We'd get so stuck in the mud we'd have to walk home."

"He liked to sit with a cat in his lap," Uncle Perry said, grinning and nudging me in the arm a little. "Maybe that's where you got your cat fever."

"Maybe it's a gene," I considered. "The cat-crazy gene. What about her?"

"She was frail," my father said. "She died of pneumonia when she was about forty-five, and then Dad married again. You knew Mamie, didn't you?"

"It was the kind of thing we could cure easily nowadays," Uncle Perry said.

My father strolled off to look at gravestones. "How do you like this one?" he called to me, and I went over to take a look. It was bright white, with sparkles shot all through it. The name was not one I knew.

"Somebody put their dirty hands all over it," Uncle Perry observed.

We walked through the cemetery toward the red brick church. There were some ancient-looking trees around it, maybe crepe myrtle, I wasn't sure, but they reminded me of the trees I used to see in Bible story books, cypress or olive, the kind Jesus sat under when he suffered the little children to come unto him.

"Good night!" I exclaimed when we had walked a little farther. "Franklin Perry Bates! Isn't that Great-Grandfather—your grandfather?" I had to consult my ancestor chart, I got all those grandfathers so mixed up.

Uncle Perry and my father came over to where I was standing. "Mary Bell Talley Bates," my uncle read out. "They were first cousins, somebody said."

"But I've never seen their graves before!" I cried. "No one ever pointed them out!"

"I guess no one ever thought of it," my father said.

·

"Where are we?" I asked. "Have I ever been on this road before?"

We were speeding along a blacktop with walls of trees on either side, covered like soft sculpture in kudzu.

"We're behind the mill," Uncle Perry said. "Slater-Marietta. I was a chemist there before I went to medical school."

"I didn't know that," I said.

My uncle Perry had had his medical office in Greenville in a long low brick building near the hospital. He was always available if Betty or I had a stomachache or fever. Once when I was thirteen, I forgot how to breathe. The more I tried to remember how it went, the harder it became to take in a breath and let it out. Each breath seemed to sit shallowly on the top of my lungs, not getting deep inside. My mother called Uncle Perry, who came right over, and listened to my chest through his stethoscope. "Well, she's aerating just fine," he said to my mother, and once he said that, I realized I was going to be okay.

Now I watched for guideposts, landmarks along the road. We were going deeper and deeper, down roads that had no names, through long stretches of woods where no houses were, across rivers that doubled back time and again, only to pop out at some familiar crossroads I could not possibly have arrived at by any compass or map. Much of the country around Marietta was still untouched, or if folks had settled there, they hadn't made much of a dent.

There were bends in the road where you might expect to come upon a band of Cherokees, or to see emancipated slaves walking out of the past. Once when I took my Grandmother Southerlin for a ride back to her old homeplace, woods where a house no longer existed, and it seemed never could have, she told me how her mother remembered a Union soldier trying their door handle as the Civil War was coming to an end. They were all hiding inside the house, and the door handle rattled and turned, but finally the soldier went away.

My father and Uncle Perry knew this territory, as my father would say, like the back of their hand. I remembered Sunday drives around Marietta, the soothing drone of my parents in the front seat as they mentioned people and places they had known, back in that mysterious time before WE were born. I recognized my father's pleasure in returning to this land, and I felt it too. I was most at home, happiest in some way I couldn't explain, riding through these woods and bottomlands and hills around Marietta. They were familiar and comforting to me in a way that had to do with blood memory.

We had come into the long narrow valley with mountains on either side called Echo Valley where my father, the oldest boy, was born. We stopped the car in the weeds on the side of the road to look at the falling-down wooden structure that had once been my father's father's general store. It was beside a small stream, where they had had a mill. My father told the story of how as a baby he was set in a big barrel of meal, and how he peed in it. It must have been warm and inviting against his bottom. My father laughed telling this story, and I stared at the old store, straining to see the past. For a moment I almost could.

"You can't possibly make that," my father said. "I wouldn't even try."

We had pulled off the main road onto a little red dirt road blocked by a metal gate. Up ahead was a steep hill with a deeply rutted road.

"Let me just see if the gate will open," Perry said.

"I'll get it," I said, jumping out. The gate swung easily, like a big metal arm opening in welcome.

"We used to come over here for church every Sunday," my father said. "When we were boys. I can't remember the last time I was here."

"We'll just go a little ways," Perry said. "If Paulette wants to see where the old church was, we can walk the rest of the way."

He gunned the motor, and we went speeding up the hill, his Chrysler at a tilt, gravel flying.

As for me I was glad we didn't have to walk. Uncle Perry carried nitroglycerine with him for his heart. He'd had angina for several years.

We stopped on a flat plateau at the top. I got out and looked around, 360 degrees. I had never seen such a pretty place. It was very quiet, and off in the distance were the Blue Ridge Mountains. Nature had taken back what humans once cleared, but through the high weeds I saw some ancient gravestones the color of rock, crooked as old teeth. There was a bird twittering in the woods, a breeze stirring the leaves, but mostly there was silence.

"We'd come here for services every Sunday," my father said. "Sometimes it was hard to get a Model T up that hill." He chuckled.

"We used to have a surrey with a fringe on top. And two white horses. One of those horses, you'd hitch him up, he'd paw the ground."

"Wanted to go!"

"We were baptized in that river," my uncle said, pointing away to the east, where one branch of the Saluda River lay obscured through the dense trees. "Submerged."

I had looked into old land deeds for the tracts of land my grandfathers and great-grandfathers had bought. The Saluda River figured prominently. The deeds were hard to read on microfiche, but were written in a beautiful script. They read, "Tract of land situated lying and being on the North Side of the middle Saluda River, running to two spruce and a pine . . ."

My father was leaning over to look at a blue flower with long spikes for petals and a round intricate center. "That's a maypop," he told me.

I couldn't remember seeing a maypop, or even thinking of one, since I was a child.

"Where would you like to go now?" Perry asked. "The old homeplace or the Bates property."

"How are y'all holding up," I asked. "I don't want to wear you out."

"No, no," my father said emphatically. "I could go all day. How 'bout you, Perry. You doing okay?"

"Let's stop at Ruth and Wade's," my uncle said. "They might be able to tell you something."

"Can I buy anybody a Coke?" I asked when we got to Marietta. It was a place in the road where three highways came together. The feed and seed store of my childhood had closed, but across the street was Marietta's answer to a mall: a Winn-Dixie, a pizza parlor, a hardware store, and a drugstore. I got us all Coca-Colas from a machine.

My uncle turned off onto another little dirt road that I recognized well. We had come to the old homeplace, where my father and his brothers grew up, on the way in to Ruth and Wade's. We stopped the car to look at it. It was a fine old two-story frame house with a gracious front porch bespeaking Southern gentility. My father's parents were considered pillars of the community. I used to fantasize, when I was a girl, that I'd buy this house back someday and live in it. But now I lived in Minneapolis, in a prairie-style stucco house.

"A young couple bought it a few years ago," my father told me. "And fixed it up real nice, I think."

The young couple had put on yellow siding, which did look nice, though I'd have preferred the house to be white, the way it used to be. They'd added a deck on the back. It looked like the kind of house that was featured in *Southern Living*, the best of the old and the new. I was surprised to see a big white duck on the deck. I didn't know if that was a touch of the old or the new.

We bounced on down the road to Ruth and Wade's. Ruth and Wade, brother and sister, were actually my mother's cousins, though they seemed more related to my father and Uncle Perry, who had lived just a shout away. When they were younger, they made their living farming the bottomland below their house, selling milk and butter from the cows they kept across Highway 288, and hauling scraps from the nearby textile mill. They had an outhouse and a junkpile bigger than their house in their red dirt yard.

We'd stop and see them on our way to our cabin at Table Rock. My mother took her old clothes to Ruth. I never saw Ruth except in men's overalls and work shoes. My mother's dresses were PTA dresses, dresses to wear to Women's Auxiliary, garden club, Circle, bridge club. But Ruth would wear the clothes to the Marietta Baptist Church. Her pale, bony face would light up—she was practically an albino. "I'm so proud to have these," she would say, holding my mother's purple Butte knit suit up to herself.

Ruth and Wade always gave us something when we left—fresh half runners, a bushel of sweet white corn, a jar of citron preserves. Ruth always gave me a pound of butter. She churned it herself and put a little molded flower on top. My mother didn't think she should give it away. "Let us pay you for it, Ruth." But Ruth would push it into my hands, saying, "No,

I'm giving it to Paulette." It would be frozen and wrapped in wax paper. My father and I loved its sweet salty taste on cornbread.

I never mentioned Ruth and Wade to any of my friends in Minneapolis. In Minneapolis I never spoke of Marietta, for how could I describe it? It was so remote from my life there, like a private revelation that couldn't be translated into words. Maybe everyone carried around in them their own past worlds, which they had had to leave behind, but which lived in them still.

My uncle tapped the horn, and Ruth came to the open screen.

"Well, Lawd, Lawd. Lawdy-me! Look who's here," she said, coming out on the porch, wiping her hands on her apron. "Paulette, my goodness. I can't tell when's the last time I laid eyes on you!"

Ruth still smelled, when I gave her a hug, of buttermilk.

We pulled up straight-back chairs in the kitchen while Ruth worked at the sink, cutting out the bad places in tomatoes Wade collected as old produce from the Winn-Dixie. Ruth had a big pot of boiling water on the wood-burning stove. "I give the slops to the pigs," she said, cutting away the bright red skin and dropping it into a colander.

"Think I might take a few of those home?" my father asked, picking up two tomatoes, and inspecting them through his bifocals.

"Daddy!" I laughed.

"Take all you want," Ruth said. "Hep yourself.

Perry, reach him a sack behind the door. Get you one, too."

It wasn't as if Daddy needed them. He had a few tomato vines himself in the narrow dirt space between his asphalt driveway and the neighbor's. But he couldn't pass up any produce.

"I've been following the drought," I said to Ruth. "I worried about how it was affecting you."

"We got in on one of them hay lifts. We keep a couple of cows over at Vannoy's. Sure was sad about H. C., Paul."

My father crossed his arms over his chest. He nodded his head, but he didn't speak.

"Wade not here?"

"He's done gone over to the mill to carry a load," Ruth said. "Maybe he'll get on back soon."

"Paulette here's working on the family tree," my father said. "If anyone can do it, Paulette can!"

"Oh, Daddy."

"Wade'd know more than I do," Ruth said. "My memory's about done for. You see this back, don't you," Ruth turned to show me. It was bent in a tortuous, unbelievable bow, where once it had been straight and strong.

"My goodness, Ruth!"

"Um, um," my father said.

"Just feel it here," Ruth said, and I put my finger tips on Ruth's back, tracing the knotty ridges of her spine. It made me think of the spines of the dinosaur skeletons I'd seen in the Science Museum in St. Paul.

"How do you stand it, Ruth?"

"Ain't nothing can be done for it," Ruth said. "Ain't that right, Perry? All them vertebra things have jumped out. Just have to live with it, I reckon."

I gave Ruth the Whitman's Sampler I had bought at the drugstore.

"Oh, oh, that does look good, Wade'll like that," she said. "But I can't eat none myself. I got that di'be-tes myself now. Sometimes I wonder how we make out."

"We better let you get your work done," my father said, rising.

"Y'all don't go!"

"We're going to take Paulette by the property," Uncle Perry said.

"Carry her on up to those old graves. Somebody said that's where some of them old Bates was buried long ago."

"Are you really going to sell the property?" I asked when we turned out of Ruth and Wade's onto Highway 276, heading north of Marietta. I had looked up the deed at the county court house. The property had been sold to my great-grandfather Franklin Perry Bates, and passed on to my grandfather and then to my father and his brothers.

"If we can get someone to buy it," my father said. "We've been trying to sell it for about ten years, and no one wants to buy it. It's not good for much. We sold off the part that had water a few years ago."

"How much land is it?"

"Ninety-six acres," my uncle and father said in unison.

"We're not going to give it away," my father confided, "but we sure would like to see a little income out of it when we could use it."

"Some fellow offered us six hundred dollars an acre but we wouldn't take it," Uncle Perry said.

This idea of them selling the old Bates property pained me. Was there something primal about hating to let go of land, or was that just something I'd learned from reading too much Southern literature? It was easy to be sentimental, nostalgic, living almost two thousand miles away, in a Northern city. What would I do with a piece of land in rural South Carolina that was all woods and no water? It was not as if we had any children—heirs, I suddenly thought of them—and even if we did (would we? would we ever, I wondered), this land would be so remote to them in experience and imagination that it would mean nothing.

We turned off the Brevard Highway onto Tilley Road, which didn't have a house on it. It was a black asphalt road, with green woods on either side. It was good dense forest, but not so thick with undergrowth that a person couldn't walk through it.

"Here's where it begins," Uncle Perry pointed out, though I could see no mark or indicator. "We sold off about fifty acres that had the spring on it."

"I don't guess the property tax is much on it," I said.

"Not much," my father mused.

My uncle stopped the car on the crest of the road. "People can see us coming either way here," he noted, though we hadn't seen a single car. We all got out.

"I'll stay here," my father said, lighting up a cigar. "I've been up that hill a million times." He blew smoke into the air and regarded it as it drifted away. I knew what he'd do while we were gone. He'd smoke his cigar and walk up the road a piece, taking in the air. I had always enjoyed being around my father. He was so at peace in the world, so much himself. How could I be his daughter, someone so busy in her mind, such a bundle of frets, desires, conflicts, fears, and longings?

"Looks like we can get across here," Uncle Perry said as we walked down the asphalt road to a level place. Uncle Perry held the rusted barbed wire fence apart for me to crawl through. Then I held it for him. We began walking up a slight incline, picking our way around fallen trees and bramble bushes. After a little while I noticed that my uncle's breathing was short.

"Should we slow down?" I asked. I pictured myself running wildly through the woods to the car for help—but there would be no help.

"This way," my uncle said, pulling back a vine for me to pass before him. "Up that little rise."

As he walked, he told me about how he and the surveyor came up here when they sold off the first fifty acres. I was beginning to wonder if we were lost. One direction seemed identical to another, and I could no longer remember which way the road was. We had been walking for about fifteen minutes, in a seemingly random way. My uncle was eighty years old, and though he always seemed totally sure of himself, totally confident, maybe we were lost in the woods. Just as I was about to question him, we came to the top of the rise, and there was a stone wall, with rocks piled to make a fence around an area the size of a small room. Everywhere were dead winter leaves. I took in at a glance that there were no gravestones. Whoever was buried in these graves was lost to time.

"When we sold this part," Uncle Perry said, "the surveyor marked off the graveyard." He pointed to red ribbons tied to a few trees in a loose circumference around the rock barrier. "You can't sell a graveyard."

We stood quietly. There was nothing to say. I had run out of questions. After a little while, I followed my uncle down the hill, back to the car.

II

6

I was standing on the corner of Fifth and Hennepin in downtown Minneapolis a few weeks after I returned from Greenville when I thought I was having a heart attack. It had only been a few days since I had had a physical, after which I had been pronounced in excellent health. But while my internist was examining me, she had lingered over my heart, and when she straightened up, I asked her anxiously what was wrong.

Oh, nothing, she said. Has anyone ever told you you have a systolic click?

Fear coursed through me. Something was wrong with my heart!

A systolic click, she explained, was no big deal. A lot of people, women especially, have them. They could come and go, which was probably why no one had ever mentioned it to me before. Nothing at all to worry about. And she had passed on to some other part of me.

That should have been the end of it, but a few days later I found myself in the downtown library, trying to read up on systolic clicks. I couldn't find anything in the medical reference books, my little click being unworthy of mention, it seemed, but as I was reading about prolapse in mitral valves, about cardiac infarction, about death, I felt such a wave of terror pass over me that I had to grab onto the chair, as if I were in an earthquake. I wandered out of the library in a daze. Knowing you're being ridiculous, even telling yourself so, isn't necessarily a deterrent. As I was standing on the corner of Fifth and Hennepin, waiting for the light to change, I noticed that my left arm was aching, and now that I thought about it, my heart was actually hurting. Was I about to drop dead of a heart attack in downtown Minneapolis? Apparently so.

Rather than cause a scene, I hurried to my car and drove home. I called Jeff at his office and asked him if he thought something could be wrong with my heart. Perhaps because he's the son of a surgeon, Jeff did not get too alarmed. When he was growing up, minor aches and pains were nothing next to the things that had to be cut out or off. He reassured me that I was okay, and I believed him, at least for a little while.

But the pain in my heart did not exactly go away. In fact, over the next few weeks, it settled into a smoldering burn in my chest, sometimes flaring up into an inferno.

I knew that time was running out for us to have a baby. But the more pressure I felt to make up my mind, the less capable I was of deciding.

It was some consolation to me that my old friend Lauren in California was just as conflicted about motherhood as I. We had visited as often as we could after I moved away, and when Lauren got married several years ago, at the age of thirty-seven, I had flown out for her wedding. Her dark hair was now salt-and-pepper. The man she married was in his mid-forties and already had three children from his previous marriage. Right away Lauren got pregnant, without intending to, and she was shocked, unnerved. She didn't feel ready (battle cry of our generation: not rea-dy!): new marriage, three stepchildren. She decided on an abortion. The doctor told her that since she had gotten pregnant so easily the first time, she wouldn't have anything to worry about if she wanted to get pregnant again.

Lauren hadn't been using birth control for some time now either, but she hadn't been able to get pregnant again. Her husband, Allen, wasn't at all sure he really wanted another child. He was nearing fifty and had spent the past twenty years raising children. But Lauren thought maybe she'd like to have a child. Only she wasn't sure. We spent hours on long distance, discussing the pros and cons of taking on an infant at our age. I would have been happy to go along in that vein forever.

But then one Sunday when we talked, she told me that she had started taking her temperature and that they were having intercourse around her ovulation. They had escalated to *trying*, doing the things you needed to do to actually get pregnant. I had a sudden vision of Lauren with a baby and pain flared in my chest. I told her good luck, but when I hung up I felt shaken. *Jeff and I were about to be left behind!*

Suddenly everyone around me was having babies, adopting, or trying to. It felt as if someone had changed the terms we were all operating under, without consulting me.

I had dinner one night with my friend Lilly, who was unmarried. In all the years I'd known her I'd never heard Lilly express the slightest interest in having a child. But now she was telling me she had already had a rubella shot, just in case.

"I'm thirty-five years old," she said intensely, "and I don't have all that much time left. I don't feel I have any control over whether I have a relationship with a man — whether I get married or not. But there's donor sperm, artificial insemination, adoption. I *know* I can have a child."

The passion with which she said this frightened me. It made me feel shaken in my own uncertainty.

But then there was my good friend Sasha. Sasha was particularly unsentimental about motherhood. She married young, had a daughter at twenty-one, and promptly got a divorce. She eventually gave up custody to her ex-husband, who was much better able to take care of Zoe than Sasha was. In the fall Zoe would be going off to Wellesley on a full scholarship. Like me, Sasha was a writer, and like me, she hadn't published a book yet. When I told her, almost bashfully, that I was thinking about trying to get pregnant, she thought I was nuts. "Why would you want to mess up your life now that you finally have it in order?"

Why indeed?

My manuscript of short stories had come back from a university press competition I had hoped to win. I tried to assess whether my book was good or bad. Some days it was good, some days bad. Clearly I was not the best person to judge.

I went back to my doctor. She assured me that the burning in my chest had nothing to do with my heart. I went home with some vague notion about my esophagus, a heretofore unconsidered body part that brought to mind a length of rubber hose such as a plumber might carry about.

One night after dinner that fall Jeff and I walked down to the local park where a neighborhood football game of thirteen-year-olds was under way. They were decked out in full uniforms with shoulder pads, which I'm sure they loved. It was amusing to see the difference in sizes at thirteen. Several shrimps were hurling themselves into the game, oblivious to getting hurt, as if scrappiness could compensate for size. To see one of those little ones attempt to tackle a big one! There was a great deal of trying to pull someone down by his jersey. The floodlights were on, and killdeers with white stripes on their wings were swooping for bugs in the piercing rays.

It was a mild October night. It had been raining, and when the boys hit, water flew. They got nice and dirty. One of the boys twisted his ankle and had to be helped to the car by his parents. Another got hit hard in midfield, and lay there as if he'd been knocked out. A few of the little yippy boys yelled "Bob! Bob!" when they saw that one of their own was fallen. Unlike some of the older boys, their voices hadn't changed. The bigger ones looked like spurts of hormones running around, conjuring up body hair, gonads, testicles. The boy really was hurt, at least in my opinion, but not a lot of fuss was made over him. He walked off, sat on the bank, and cried. Tears filled my eyes. A woman—his mother or another player's mother—came over, stooped down, and comforted him. Later, a few men came by and kind of patted him on the shoulder. Everybody pretty much left him alone until he had time to get over it. Later we saw that he had gotten up and rejoined the players on the side.

Out on the field the mixture of boys jumbled into each other on slow runs. The score was twenty-four to zip, and there were a lot of interceptions and fumbles. Once when a small boy punted a short squirt, another player on his team kicked the ball farther. When the coach on the other side of the field yelled "Execution, gentleman, execution," everyone on the sidelines laughed. Meanwhile, the children moved in slow motion, miniature men on the park field under the bright lights.

We were standing next to a mother who was watching her son play, with a good deal of apprehension. He was a nice-sized kid, but she told us she didn't want him to play, and he didn't want to, but peer pressure and all that . . . I thought how hard it must be to be a parent. How much was involved! What a tremendous feat it was. To have a child was to be at such risk. Every day the news was full of stories of children dying of cancer, abducted and missing, falling under the school bus wheels, not to mention the minor catastrophes that accompanied growing up. To have a child was to open yourself forever to possible heartache. No wonder I was afraid to do it.

I looked around at the other parents standing on the sidelines watching the game. It occurred to me that everyone had children; that was what people *did*, the natural order of things. Of course I knew that not everyone had children. Plenty of people didn't. Where were they? I was beginning to feel out of the mainstream, channeled into a side eddy of life. It set up a deep uneasiness in me to think that I might be *different*. At a deep level I felt that having children was what I was supposed to do.

The problem was, I had come to question anything I was *supposed* to do, especially as a woman. That was the legacy of my generation, a habit I couldn't break. I was always afraid society was trying to put one over on me, which usually it was. I didn't know what to make of this growing interest in having a child, except that it was charged with an amazing amount of ambivalence, conflict, desire, and confusion. Did I really want to be a mother, or did I really just want to conform to society's expectations for me? And how could I separate my own true self from what I had incorporated growing up in a society where motherhood was such an assumption? I had been struggling to be conscious, to have control over my life, to make decisions rather than "go along," so how could I give the reins over to something as big and unconscious and powerful as maternal instinct? The little life I had been constructing would be gobbled up. The maternal instinct waiting to be unleashed in me might turn out to be like the plant in *Little Shop of Horrors*.

"How are you feeling about it these days?" I asked Jeff as we walked home in the dark.

"I don't know," he said. "I haven't been thinking about it.

How could he not think about it! I thought about it all the time now. Nights when we were lying in bed, wandering near to sleep, I'd suddenly say, *Maybe we're making a terrible mistake not to have a child. Maybe we really should be trying!* After a few more moments, I'd say, *But maybe it would be a terrible — a terrible! — mistake to have a child. What do you think?*

But Jeff, who is incapable of thinking of life as a series of pitfalls, would already be asleep.

I'd lie awake then, counting up the dangers. In

the netherworld between waking and sleep, I feared that if we did want a child, we wouldn't be able to have one; or if I did conceive, I'd have a miscarriage. Maybe the baby would be stillborn, or I'd die in labor. And then there was always motherhood itself, being swallowed up by caretaking, becoming a complete stranger to myself. I worried about colic, harelip, sudden infant death syndrome, spina bifida. I worried that the child would grow up to be an intractable alienated teenager who would break Jeff's heart and mine. I feared we'd give birth to a born-again Christian or a Republican . . .

"But why do you think it is," I pressed on now, "that we've never had a child? Why is it, do you think, that in all these years together, we've never managed to do it?"

"We haven't been together all that long," he tried.

"Ten years! I mean, is there something wrong with us? Together, I mean. What is it? We've been together ten years, married for six. Where has it gone? And why didn't we think of having a child earlier? We never actually did, you know. We were the children, I suppose."

"As I recall you never wanted a child before," Jeff said. "And anyway, it took us a while to get together, and then there was law school, and then moving back here, trying to get established, me getting a job, you working and writing. All that. These things take time. We weren't really thinking about children much before."

"But doesn't it bother you? Do you ever feel bad about it?"

He considered this for a moment.

"Not bad. I guess I've just been playing the cards life dealt me. I'm not sure we're totally in control."

It was so different for Jeff and me. Fatherhood was not the loaded issue for him that motherhood was for me.

"I feel so troubled," I said. I shook my head. "Having a child. The simplest thing in the world, you'd think. But I don't know whether I want to change in that way. And the thing is, it's probably too late!"

We were silent for awhile, trudging along. "Would it make it easier if we just laid the whole thing to rest?" Jeff asked. "What if I decided—what if I took the responsibility for the decision—and said that I didn't want to have a child. How would that make you feel?"

"Is that what you really want?"

"I don't know," he said. "Sometimes it is and sometimes it isn't. Most people don't really question it, you know. They just know they want children or assume they do, without really giving it much thought, or they just get pregnant before they're ready. I don't think it's going to work out that way for us, though. We're not spring chickens, you know. I don't think we need a child to be happy. I mean, we *are* happy. At least I am."

"You are?" I said, surprised. "Thank goodness." I

was beginning to feel that I was going to be unhappy either way.

"I don't necessarily always want to practice law," Jeff said. "But if we have a child, we'll have to be worrying about putting him—her—it—through college when we're sixty-five. I don't know that we want to take it all on at this point in our lives."

I was silent for a while. "I can't believe how this whole issue upsets me. What really gets me is that I may not be able to get pregnant. It's funny, isn't it? I'm not sure I really want a kid now, but when I think I might *never* have one, I feel"—the word caught in my throat—"bereft."

We had come to the front porch. We stopped to stomp our boots. I caught a glimpse of Jeff's face, and there was a look on it. It wasn't about having or not having a child. It was about me.

"So let's have one," Jeff said.

I gave a mournful snort. Have one, not have one, it didn't seem to matter what got said. Words. We were full of them. We were both actually pretty good at them. But whatever it was inside me that was battling it out was not amenable to words.

That night I dreamed I had a baby. It was a very tiny baby, but in the distortion that is natural to dreams, I took it for granted. But then the baby started to disappear. It began to dissolve back into a kind of white froth, like protoplasm. All I could find of it was a thicker, clearer blob that beat like a heart. But it was nothing that resembled a baby any more.

·

The pain in my chest did not go away. In fact, my symptoms escalated over the fall to include my stomach. I had never thought much about my stomach before. It had always worked so quietly and efficiently, like a good dishwasher. But now it made itself known. I could feel it there inside me, irritated, agitated, off its cycle, out of control. Now I never knew what strange thing it was going to do. It went into reverse sometimes, mainly at night, when I was lying down. Gravity was against me. Or it made angry sounds, like a creaking door in a haunted house. I was wildly hungry at odd times, or strangely full, as if things had stuck in my craw. Once when we were driving in the country, it felt exactly as if land mines were being detonated inside me. Get me to a hospital quick, I told Jeff. Instead he got me a carton of milk, which eased somewhat the horrible sensations.

I went in for a stomach X-ray and was relieved to hear that I did not have an ulcer. My doctor was reassuring. This thing would run its course. In the meantime, she recommended antacids. I had never had an antacid in my life, but suddenly I saw that the whole economy turned on them: Maalox, Milanta, Riopan Plus, Gelusil. It was a litany with which I would become well acquainted. Now when ads came on TV showing sponges soaking up stomach acid, I was all eyes.

I began taking my temperature, as I had read about in *Fertility Awareness*, charting it in tenths of degrees with a basal thermometer on a graph I had gotten from my gynecologist's office. I wanted to find out if I was even ovulating. When my temperature actually rose five-tenths of a degree on the fourteenth day, a sign that I was probably ovulating, I was excited. The next month I told Jeff that I thought maybe we ought to try to cover my fertile period, just to see what would happen, so we had intercourse for five days in a row. At first Jeff was wildly enthusiastic, but by the fifth day, some of the thrill was gone. He had trouble getting it up, a first and hopefully last for him, and when he finally did manage to get inside me, I couldn't help but laugh. That made him mad, but then he started laughing too, and in the end, the sperm just sort of drizzled out. "That," he said as he lay beached on top of me, "is about as close as two people can come to artificial insemination."

But I didn't get pregnant. In a way I hadn't expected to, but on the other hand, I absolutely had. And now there was no getting around that we were actually *trying*.

Every day when I wasn't teaching, I sat at my desk and wrote. All I knew for sure was that when I wasn't writing, I was miserable. I didn't really see how I could have a baby and do this work. It didn't faze me that other women did. I felt that I was an either-or sort of person, someone who could do either motherhood or writing "right"—but not both of them. I was someone who had to choose. But for all my talk about choices, I was afraid to make them, because choosing meant giving something up.

I had to wrestle with the heebie-jeebies of writing. I didn't know if I'd ever accomplish anything or not. There were a million different directions a thing could take off in, and I wasn't sure if any one of them was right. Sometimes I didn't know if what I was working on was a short story or a novel. I only knew that whatever it was, it was going to take a hell of a lot of work, months and months, and maybe even years. And then I had no idea if it would be published. I wondered if I was fooling myself.

One day I wrote down all the shoulds that filled my head: *I should write snappy, witty, currently hip stories; I should lead another kind of life, such as that of a single (divorced?) woman in New York so that I have snappy, witty, acerbic, lonely things to write about; I should write politically important stuff, about nuclear threat especially; I should be very fancy with language—style is everything; I should not write autobiographical stuff, especially about my father and mother; I should know what I'm doing; I should be more productive; I should be further along; I should be an expert; I should have learned more craft in all these years of trying; I should try harder; I shouldn't try so hard; I should be better read; I should be more articulate and interesting; I should be more sophisticated and dismiss a lot of what I read as crap; I should promote my writing more, be more aggressive somehow—how? I should know. I should write real fiction — made-up stuff about made-up people. I should "turn elusive feelings into shimmering stories that possess the power both to charm and move us." I should be charming and moving. I should be more social. I should stay home more and write. I should write before allowing myself treats — like lunch. I should make a list of all the crazy shoulds in my head so I could once and for all replace them with statements like "I am gentle with myself."*

That night I woke up in a cold sweat. It came to me that if I didn't publish a book soon, in the next year or two, if I didn't finally accomplish what I had been trying to do for so long, I would surely die. I didn't know what form this death would take, but a death it would be nonetheless.

What had started as an ache in my arm and a pain in my chest had developed into constant, pervasive stomach trouble. A few days before Christmas I found myself in a flimsy hospital gown, lying on my side while a gastroenterologist directed me to swallow a tube so he could look inside my stomach. I didn't even mind. I was so upset with the state of my health that I just wanted to know what was wrong. I had lost my previous springy identity, and turned into someone wrapped around a painful esophagus and stomach, someone whose whole life had been taken over by worry and pain. This, I knew, was what could happen to people in life. It was happening to me. I gagged a little but mainly I cooperated. I swallowed the thing right down and let his big eye take a look.

While I was recovering from the sedative, the doctor came in to talk to us. He hadn't found anything too bad, he said. No cancer. No ulcer. Just a little redness in the esophagus and stomach lining. A little redness! All this, and a little redness? I could hardly believe my ears. Well, what is going on? I implored him. What *is* wrong with me? And why?

Oh, he said, laughing lightly. You're probably just going through a midlife crisis.

7

It would be funny — if it weren't so painful — how up until about the age of twenty-one the worst mistake a girl like me could make would be to have a baby before she got married, and then almost overnight the worst mistake became to get married and have a baby — both of which I had avoided. I had always been one to want to be in control, never to make a mistake. But now I was beginning to wonder if maybe I wasn't about to make — if I hadn't already — the biggest mistake of all: I was about to miss out on having a child.

How to explain this? I found myself thinking back to my years in California in the early seventies, when it seemed that all I had assumed and expected growing up was being challenged, over-turned, thrown out like my panty girdle. Marriage, once the bedrock of a woman's life, now seemed like a dirty trick, a dangerous trap you'd be smart to avoid. As if to verify what was in the air, back home in South Carolina, my own sister and her husband were getting a divorce. Betty had done things the way we had been raised, and now everything she had believed in and counted on was kaput. *Virgin-wife-divorcée.*

The thing was, when I thought about that time, what I remembered was being obsessed with men. I didn't want to marry, exactly. True to the times, I viewed marriage with skepticism and disdain. I viewed *men* with skepticism and disdain, even as I was attracted to them. Men had become associated in my mind with the thwarting of my own ambitions. But I couldn't stay away from them.

By 1971 I was living alone in the woods in a little cabin in Portola Valley. Stanford had hired me as a Jones Lecturer to teach creative writing, which I would do for the next three years. I was teaching and writing, and if my love life left something to be desired, I had many wonderful women friends who were trying, like me, to make up new lives for themselves, lives for which we did not have a pattern.

It was during these years that I met Lauren. Lauren lived in a little cabin over the ridge from my own cabin in Portola Valley. I had met her one day when I was driving back to my cottage from campus. She was hitchhiking on Alpine Road, and I picked her up in my Volkswagen camper. I had seen her around campus—her dark curly hair in an Afro, lots of turquoise jewelry, a certain sophistication and savoir faire that meant she was from the East Coast. She had gone to Vassar and now was working as a secretary on campus, having dropped out of graduate school. When we arrived at her place, she invited me in. It was even smaller than my own cabin and had the same funky, knowing style that Lauren had. There were pillows and curtains she had made from beautiful fabrics, baskets of unusual textures and shapes, exotic plants, and a sullen-looking boyfriend named Ron.

Ron was as close as I had gotten to an actual hippie. His hair was long and stringy blond, he played the guitar, he didn't work or go to school, and he smoked a lot of dope. Lauren, like me, was basically middle class, attracted to the ideals of the sixties, but finding it hard to deal with an actual embodiment of them. She and Ron were in the process of breaking up.

My lover at the time was an undergraduate whose boyish charms were irresistible, at least to me. With Mark I thought I could take on the role of the older, more experienced woman (I was three years older) who thought love was nice, but not the total conflicted obsession it actually was for me. When he took me at my word, and began sleeping around, I was crushed. I could never quite make the Carolina part of me keep up with the California part.

Lauren and I would hike the mile or so through the eucalyptus woods between our cabins to cook whole wheat macaroni and cheese in her big earthenware pot or teriyaki chicken on my hibachi grill out back. We'd drive over to the coast for the day, go to lectures and readings together, have dinner parties for our friends, call each other nearly every day. The sight of Lauren with her halo of dark hair and her bright Guatemalan poncho as she strode up the dirt road to my place always filled me with joy.

Once we tried to be lovers, hoping we could be for each other all that we found so lacking in men. But curling against each other in our flannel nightgowns, we could not arouse the necessary passion. This was not the hot lesbian love we had hoped for, but more like the slumber parties we had attended as girls, with the same degree of giggling.

Lauren had a big black lab named Smoker, and I had my cat, Charlotte. These were our children. The animals were happy to indulge us, lapping up all that mother-love. But one summer Lauren and I went to Mexico, and I left Charlotte with some students who were house-sitting my cottage. When I got home to South Carolina, I called my own number in California, and learned that Charlotte had died. She had died almost immediately after I had left, within a few days. I sat on my parents' bed and received the blow. It was a contagious virus, the student said, and there was nothing the vet could do. But I knew why Charlotte had died. I had left her and the invisible thread that ran between us had been broken.

I didn't get another cat for quite some time. I couldn't replace Charlotte. But then one day another cat appeared on my back steps in Portola Valley, this one small and black, pathetic, starved, half-wild. Unable to help myself, I began to put food out for it.

And of course, predictably, it showed up not long after with three kittens in tow: black ones, babies with yellow eyes.

But what to do? I couldn't just keep feeding them, for then there would be more and more wild cats in the woods. I was applying for teaching jobs, and next year, if I was lucky, I'd be hired someplace. I'd be leaving Portola Valley. Then who would feed them? I decided on a plan. I would trap them and tame them, and after that . . . I didn't really know. Mainly, I had a deep longing to get my hands on them, to make them my own.

I began moving the food that I placed on the back steps closer and closer to the door, finally putting it inside the house so that the cat and kittens had to come in to get it. They did so warily at first, with the greatest trepidation, but I was silent, patient, still. Hadn't I learned that from cats? After a few days, when no harm befell them, they let down their guard a little. I moved the food farther in and they couldn't help themselves, they came to it. Finally one day, while they were eating, I ran around the house and slammed the back door to trap them inside. One kitten and the mother were fast enough to escape, and I never saw them again. But now I had two wild black kittens trapped inside my house.

It took a long time. I didn't try to rush it. They bit and scratched every time I caught them, but I made a point of touching them once a day: no more, no less. They fled to any hiding spot they could jam themselves into, under, or between. My hands were covered with scratches. Sometimes I'd simply sit quietly, and watch them venture out. I took my time. I had plenty of patience. I caught them once a day, then let them go, to prove they could be touched by me and live. They ate my food and gradually they got used to my giant feet, my giant hands, my giant face.

They developed a taste for creature comforts. They discovered the top of my bed with its big soft quilt. And one day when I sat down at my desk to write, one of them was curled in the metal basket that held my papers, under the warmth of the desk light. He did not flee. He stayed put, though I saw that it took all his nerve. I reached out my hand, ever so slowly. The kitten regarded the approach of this hand with wide eyes, crouching a little, but he did not run away. My index finger reached him, and with that one finger, very delicately, I stroked his shiny black fur, each hair a separate wonder of light under the bright lamp. Then slowly, carefully, I withdrew my finger. I picked up my pen and began to write.

I named them Cecil and Creepy, and that first year of their childhood was rather traumatic. I was used to Charlotte, her maturity, and these were kids, these were brats, running at top speed over the back of the couch, sharpening their sprouting claws on my curtains, leaping from counter to table top, wrestling with each other at all hours of the night, scrambling around corners and leaping into the air with mock fight or fright. But if I missed a good night's sleep, I didn't mind too much. I was twenty-seven years old, a long way from home, in love with the wrong man, afraid of marriage, uncertain about the future, out on a limb, trying to make something of myself.

The man I was in love with was named Pete, and he was living with a friend of mine named Sondra. They had cats, too—two delicate Burmese. He was already committed, cat-wise, but ambivalent, woman-wise.

It had started like this: One day he left a note in my mailbox asking if he could meet me for coffee at the student union. The romantic thought crossed my mind that he wanted to tell me he loved me. More likely, he wanted to talk about Sondra. I was in a women's group with Sondra and I knew from her that their relationship was not a happy one. Pete was a moody man, from a sad background; his father had been an alcoholic and had abandoned the family when Pete was a child. There was something arrested and childlike about Pete, something vulnerable and poignant that cried out to be saved.

So there we were sitting in the union having coffee when he told me he was in love with me. "I've given it a lot of thought," he said (he was a Ph.D. candidate, the brainy type), "and it's you I love, not Sondra. In fact, I think you may be the only person I can ever love."

I was shocked and flattered, always pleased to have anyone fall in love with me. "But Pete," I said delicately, "what about Sondra? You're already taken." Something he himself seemed to forget.

"I needed to tell you," he said. "I need you to know." He had a big nose and small hands. I felt like laughing. The very idea was so ludicrous, preposterous! I wasn't even attracted to him, not that that would matter, I told myself quickly. Sondra was my friend, my "sister." I wasn't about to get involved with the likes of Pete.

Still, often after that, whenever I'd come out of the English department building, there he'd be, sitting on a bench in the courtyard. I knew he wanted to see me. He liked to watch me. He was like a mirror, and as I'd walk away from him, I'd see myself reflected as my most desired image, that of a desirable woman.

One day Pete drove up to my cottage in Portola Valley. He wanted to talk.

"You're not like Sondra," he said. "It's as if Sondra and I are already middle aged, as if we've been married for twenty years. But there's something untamed about you. You want to be a writer. You're such a free spirit."

Free spirit! I had to snort. But on the other hand, why not? I tried it on for size.

"But Sondra's a wonderful person," I argued. "She so—so *good*." I made it sound dull. I thought of the apartment they rented, the home they had together, where I had been to dinner parties several times. It was filled with little domestic touches, handmade curtains of dark blue print, a round oak table they had bought and refinished, a couple-coziness that had, at times, made me feel lonely. But not right now. Now I was seeing myself as Pete saw me, a sexual, independent, free woman. Let Sondra be the wife-type, I would be the lover-type. I felt a swell of what I should have recognized as hubris.

Not too long after that, Pete sent me a dozen roses. Lauren was coming to dinner that night, and I didn't tell her about them. I hid them in a closet. That was the moment when I became implicated. Nothing external had changed, nothing had happened, but I had crossed over. Pete and I were often around each other, at dinner parties or in the English department, and now those meetings were charged with an illicit energy. No one else knew what had passed between us, and the private knowledge of his attraction was in every glance, in every conversation. The fact that we didn't act only intensified the situation.

We became lovers. So much for sisterhood. I had built the case in my mind that it wasn't wrong, that we should be together, that I could handle it. I wanted to test my newfound power, the power to be the independent woman I wanted to be, and also to have a lover. And of course, predictably, not too long after we became lovers, Pete began to vacillate. He was afraid to make a complete break with Sondra. And his uncertainty, once I had committed my-self, was the perfect hook for pulling me deeper in.

He loved me, he didn't love me, he loved me, he didn't love me. Summer was finally at an end, and what was more, I had been offered a job, a good job, sort of, a renewable one-year visiting assistant professorship teaching creative writing at the University of Minnesota. I would move to Minneapolis. We three were all leaving California anyway: Pete, Sondra, me. I hugged Lauren good-bye for now and then I drove across the country in my Volkswagen camper full of cats and plants. Pete had said he would come to me, but in the meantime, I was on my own. Cecil and Creepy were not happy about traveling. But what else could I do? They were not the sort of cats I could just give away. Once wild kittens, always wild cats, the vet had told me when I took them in for psychoanalysis. They loved me, me alone, and I would take care of them. I took them with me to Minneapolis, a new city where I knew no one, and where I would be waiting for Pete to come to me. They need me, I said to myself.

I checked into a seedy motel room in Brooklyn Center on the outskirts of Minneapolis because it would take cats. My room had a cheap formica desk with three drawers on one side, an oversized lamp, a sagging bed, and a sickening orange-colored armchair. During the days I looked for a place to live. I did not want to show my face at the university, to meet the department chair and the other professors. They could wait to find out they had made a mistake. I was feeling so displaced, disoriented. I was waiting for Pete to come help me.

Pete arrived, and it was not as I had hoped. At night he got up after we had gone to bed and sat in the orange chair, drinking and brooding. I didn't know what to say. I didn't know how to make him happy.

"I'm not sure you want to marry and have children," Pete said to me. "And Sondra does. I want to have children. I see it as a way to redeem my own childhood."

What was going on here? I got the feeling he wanted to turn me into another Sondra, someone to take care of him, cook his meals, have his babies while he had his career. Then, I reasoned, he'd go out and find another me, someone whom he saw as a sexy, independent, artistic type he could complain to.

But the idea that he might not love me, that he might *leave* me, if I didn't want to marry and have children—*if I couldn't say for sure, right then*—tortured me. I had finished a novel, but I knew it was probably not going to be published. I needed time to develop as a writer, and I had the feeling that marriage—at least in the near future and at least to Pete—would not exactly further my own goals.

"Look," he said, "I do love you. But I love Sondra, too. She's been so good to me. And she wants children. I'm not sure you do."

But what about what I might want? I thought. *Why is this so much about you?*

We were staying at the motel while I searched for the perfect apartment for my perfect life with Pete. But finally I realized I would just have to take a place, any place, that was all there was to it. I rented an ugly furnished apartment in an ugly brownstone near campus because it allowed cats. By the time I moved in Pete was gone. He went back to Stanford, saying he had to finish some work, but I knew he was trying to make up his mind between Sondra and me.

Slowly, slowly, life settled down. I settled down. I began my teaching job at the university, and it was all right. It was fine. All the pieces of myself, which had been strewn around so by Pete, were coalescing again. At night I sat on the couch—nubby brown, made of some synthetic material with gold threads in it—with Cecil and Creepy, and we watched TV with the glazed look of survivors.

One evening a month or so after I moved in, Pete called to say that he wanted to come back to me. He wanted to come live with me. "I love you," he said. "It's you I really love." We took that word very seriously: love. What I needed to do, he said, was find a better place for us to live.

It was about this time that Cecil did not return

one day after I had let him out. I had been reluctant at first to let the cats out. But they were California cats, used to being outside, longing for dirt and grass. For a while I would sit on the landing to watch them. They ventured a little farther away every day—but they always came back.

Only this time Cecil didn't. Where was he? I called and called, I walked around the block, I passed the night in a restless sleep, getting up often to check at the back door. In the morning he was not there, nor the next, nor the next. I visited the pound, I ran a notice in Lost and Found, I looked compulsively out the window every few minutes when I was home. But he was gone, gone.

I found a new apartment, available on the first of the year. It was not a perfect place—I was afraid Pete wouldn't like it—but when I described it to him over long distance, he sounded pleased. I told him how Cecil was missing, but I didn't go into the details, how I tried, lying in bed at night, to find him in my imagination. To imagine his fate. Where was he? In someone's house? Cecil would never let anyone touch him; no one but me. He must have been hit by a car or killed by a dog. The worst thought was that he was lost, running through the big city as winter was coming on, trying to find his way back to me.

November passed, and no sign of him. Then one evening, when I was waiting for a ride in front of my building, very far away, I heard him calling. He was calling and calling, but how could it be Cecil? It was surely some other cat, but the calling came closer, moved toward me, and then I saw him, my own black streak, crossing the corner in a low running crouch, coming toward me, calling and calling my name. The sound of his voice! He had no vocabulary, he had no range—but what feeling he managed to convey in those sounds. He was coming back! I swooped him up, knowing the exact size and weight of his body. I rushed him inside, where he and Creepy sniffed each other, and then he settled down on my bed and fell asleep. I locked the door behind me and met my friend out front. And all evening, as we went to dinner and a play, I had an incredible feeling of happiness, that Cecil had come home.

Pete did not come back. He called me the night before he was scheduled to arrive, the night before we were to move to the new apartment, and told me he had gone back to Sondra.

It was perfect timing, I had to hand it to him. Well, I liked the new apartment and besides I had put down the first and last month's rent to hold it. I moved in with Cecil and Creepy to the top of a duplex near a large grain elevator, still within walking distance of campus. It was not a place with any "street appeal." It was a rectangular, absolutely plain box with a flat roof, an upstairs, a downstairs, painted white, with some pink trim. It was the most anonymous, utilitarian-looking place I had ever seen, but it was home. I began to acquire, here and there, my own furniture, a couch from Goodwill, a bedstead discovered at a garage sale, a lamp from a used furniture store. And over time, the wound that was Pete began to heal.

8

"... soothing, loving, healing energy."

I was lying on the floor with my hands folded across my chest. My mouth was open, as if my jaw was unhinged. The blinds were pulled, and even though it was the middle of the afternoon it was dark in the room.

It was January now, and I had set my fortieth birthday in May as the deadline for giving up on having a child. We were *trying* all right, me taking my temperature and us having intercourse around the right time. But nothing was happening.

"Now call the energy back up into that part of your body that needs special attention, and let the soothing, loving, healing energy caress and nurture that part of your body. Say to yourself, 'I love this part of my body. I appreciate it.'"

Bob Griswold's voice—the voice on the tape—was oddly soothing, mainly, I thought, because it was so plain, so Midwestern. The first time I put the tape on, I almost laughed out loud. I had expected someone putting out "Love Tapes" to be California hip, guruish, and Bob Griswold—even his name!—

was so unhip. The image his voice conjured up was not some ectomorphic bearded type in love beads, but rather an average guy in a brown suit, with a white shirt of some slightly silky substance. Someone who grew up in Sioux City, Iowa, or Grand Forks, North Dakota; someone totally lacking in a sense of irony. It was this quality—that he seemed incapable of taking an ironic stance toward life— that I found so appealing.

Jeff had laughed ruefully the first time he heard the tape, but then he wasn't having stomach trouble. It was a mistake to play it for him—one I hadn't made since. I listened to it when I was alone: stolen moments with Bob Griswold, almost as if he were a lover. A lover of soothing, loving, healing energy.

Now there were sounds of waves in the background, and Bob was telling me to imagine that I was standing at the seashore. But instead I thought about how I was almost forty and I didn't have a book or a baby. My stomach released a burst of acid. If I didn't get pregnant by forty, I told myself, I would give up. Forty was too old. Wasn't it? It certainly sounded old to me. I had to face it, I told myself, I had to come to terms with not having a child. Unless I had one, that is.

I tried to concentrate again on the tape. "Now imagine a ball of light that you hold in your hands . . . a ball of purest energy . . ." I imagined instead Bob Griswold in a small sound room removing the needle from the record of waves. How anyone could sit there with a straight face and tell you to imagine holding a ball of energy in your hands! But I tried. I really did. I wanted to, as Bob put it, program myself for better health. I needed help. I tried with all my might to relax.

But now my mind was wandering into a new minefield, that of Jeff's job. He was an associate at a small law firm, and in the past few months there had been a lot of talk of him making partner. Making partner was supposed to be a good thing, but unfortunately Jeff wanted out. He had an independent streak that made him want to get away from all the hassles involved in the firm. Maybe it ran in his family; both his father and grandfather, doctors, had worked for themselves. Lately he was talking about quitting his job and going on his own, solo—an idea that both enticed and scared the pants off of us.

You are now in a much deeper, more relaxed state of being, Bob intoned.

In February my mother had a radical mastectomy. In a routine mammogram, they had found a tiny spidery spot of cancer. When my father called to tell me the diagnosis, I sat on the landing of the stairs, holding the phone to my ear with a complete sense of disbelief. Nothing had ever been wrong with my mother and as far as I was concerned, nothing *could* be wrong with her. She had never been sick, never showed any sign of weakness. I was filled with so much shock and fear that I felt light-headed and dizzy.

She wanted the breast removed immediately and so the operation was scheduled for the next day. When I flew to Greenville that weekend, I found my mother in a pale blue bed jacket in her hospital bed recovering from the operation and in good spirits. "I made up my mind that getting rid of the breast was the price of living," she said to me, "and I was glad to pay it." The cancer hadn't spread to her lymph nodes, which meant her prognosis was good.

I enjoyed visiting my mother at the hospital. I needed to be with her, to partake of her, to do for her. In a few days I had gone from thinking she was going to die to believing her life had been saved. It was a lifesaving operation, the woman who visited new mastectomy patients told us. She was living proof herself. She showed my mother exercises such as crawling her fingers up the wall to strengthen the affected side, and showed us breast prostheses matter-of-factly. My mother was realistic and practical, and I felt a tremendous relief that we had been spared this time.

One day while I was visiting her, a favorite nurse she had made friends with came in. My mother greeted her affectionately, and reached out warmly to take the nurse's hand. I was taken by surprise, suddenly seeing my mother as a stranger might see her, someone gracious and endearing. I was so used to guarding against my mother, protecting myself from her. At that moment I felt jealous. I wished that my relationship to my mother could be as simple and easy as that nurse's.

My mother had always seemed so powerful to me, a force that would take me over if I allowed it. When I thought of her, the image that came to mind was her big Buick. My mother had always had a Buick, to me the perfect symbol of her authority when I was growing up. When I thought of her, I pictured her wheeling around in her big car, picking me up at school, or pulling into our attached garage and honking the horn for Betty and me to come unload the groceries.

Every day during my visit, I drove home from the hospital in her current Buick, a twelve-year-old model I maneuvered through traffic as if I were steering the QEII. My father and I settled in peacefully together, puttering around the house, watching TV, and cooking down-home Southern meals between hospital visits. My father and I got along like bread and butter; I never felt in combat with him the way I sometimes did with Mother. But of course he had never had to enter the fray. He had gone off to work every day when we were growing up and left Mother with the difficult job of molding us into acceptable human beings.

I sometimes thought that if I could be the father, I'd have no hesitation about wanting a child. Being the father meant you got to enjoy your offspring, while being the mother meant constant travail. I didn't mean the physical hard work of tending a child, though that was nothing to sneeze at. I meant the burden of being totally responsible for the socialization of a fledgling. When I thought of my own mother, I didn't think of her pleasure in us (I knew she loved us, though that seemed, in some ways, the least of it) but of her endless diligence in directing and shaping us. It made me tired just to think of it; something in me shrank from taking it on.

I had never thought very much about my mother's influence on my own views of motherhood, perhaps because I hadn't had to. But of course I had "learned" what a mother was at her knee. Had what I had absorbed about motherhood from her made me not want to do it? By not becoming a mother, had I been, in effect, rejecting my own mother's life?

No wonder I envied that nurse. My own relationship to Mother seemed so complex and deep that I had trouble knowing where to start, how to get a foothold on understanding it.

Once when we were driving through Marietta on the way to our cabin, my mother had teased our father about a former girlfriend of his named Bessie, who had lived in a little white mill house, right on the highway, that we saw every time we passed by. It had a porch swing and a plaster of Paris duck and a row of little white ducklings in the front yard. I understood that Bessie was country and that she was fat. My mother was saying, in effect, that she had saved my father from Bessie. Lucky for my father that he had married Mother, so slim and pretty, so nice and citified, being from Texarkana and all.

Long after my mother and father had forgotten about Bessie, I continued to think of her. I knew just what she was like, even though I never saw her: a big moon face, upper arms that shimmied, a body under her cotton dress that spread like a river over-flowing its banks. Bessie wouldn't be concerned with the millions of things my mother cared about: if my clothes were ironed, if I wore braces to correct my snaggletooth, if I practiced the piano an hour a day. I liked to thrill and scare myself with the idea that my father might actually have married Bessie and then she would be my mother. We'd live in Marietta, and I'd be little Bessie, or rather big little Bessie. I'd be fat and I'd be country. This thought—that my mother and all her influence disappear from my life—filled me with deep longing and something approaching terror.

When we were children, her competence and authority anchored our world. She was clearly the Mama, who knew all and did all. We needed her so completely, and she was always there for us. It never would have occurred to me that she wouldn't have been where she'd said she'd be at a certain time, or that she wouldn't volunteer to be homeroom mother or to carry a load of my classmates to a skating party in her big Buick. She monitored our homework, dressed us in precious outfits, fed us well-balanced meals, bought us Barbie dolls and hula hoops when they were the fad, let us lounge in bed with maga-zines and ginger ale when we were sick, requested the best teachers for us, rubbed Solarcaine on our sunburns, gave us surprise birthday parties, took us to piano and ballet lessons, taught us our manners. I was always proud of her beauty parlor hair, her handsome suits, her certainty about what to do. As a child I had regarded her with a profound, amazed gratitude, for how could I have survived without her?

But the other side of all this competence was control. We were a little afraid of her as children, though we accepted this as natural, her right as the Mama, part of her power and authority that we counted on. Betty and I were capable of running wild, acting up, and sometimes we asked for it. Those times when we had gone too far she'd make us pick a switch from the big green bush out the back door, and she'd switch the backs of our legs until red lines appeared. We were unlikely to jump up and down screaming on our beds again, or fight with one another until one of us went crying to Mama. It got to where we took it for granted that we'd do what pleased her, what she wanted us to do. We were able to read her signals, her looks, one word, and there was no longer any need for switches.

We existed, then, between intense dependence on our mother and resentment that she had so much power. As long as we were little girls, this combination of our need and her control worked pretty well, but Betty and I couldn't be children forever. We had to grow up. By the time we were teenagers the very qualities in her we had valued in childhood became the source of conflict. We began to resist her, to resent her, to separate from her, the normal thing. But this pulling apart was not without its pain, anger, and sorrow on both sides.

I can mark the specific moment when my relationship with my mother shifted. It was the spring of seventh grade, that year when so much else was changing. We started dating in the seventh grade in Greenville, with the boys' fathers chauffeuring us around. At parties we'd go on "proms" where we'd walk around the block in couples to escape the chaperones. At this particular party I'm remembering I went on a prom with Tommy Cantrell, whom I liked, and who liked me. At one point, under the big canopy of an evergreen tree that branched out over the sidewalk, he put his hand on my arm to stop me. There in the dark he kissed me, sweetly, tenderly, on the cheek. We commenced walking again. Not a word was said. But I had been kissed, my first kiss, and I felt brand new, loved.

When I got home, my mother was waiting for me, as she waited for me every time, and as usual, we sat on the ledge of the fireplace in the den so I could tell her about the party. I must have told her everything back then, which seems odd, for during so much of my life I kept a lot from her. I began to tell her about the party, and then about walking around the block with Tommy Cantrell. Something in me hesitated as I approached the kiss, but I was accustomed to telling her everything. I was not yet clear on where she stopped and I started. So I told her how Tommy had kissed me. Where, she asked, and I told her on the cheek. Then she said, "And did you give him a peck back?"

Peck? Everything in me shrunk. She was making fun of my precious kiss. I knew she didn't mean anything by it, really. But that was just the point. To her I was still a little girl talking about getting a peck on the cheek from a little boy. How I wished I could take that part back! I felt myself recoil from my mother. I understood that from then on I would not be telling her everything. I looked back at her from across a gulf.

It's hard for me to separate my sense of my mother when I was growing up from the society we existed in back then, Greenville in the fifties and early sixties. The Greenville of my girlhood was amazingly complex and rigid, with well-established social class and racial rules, as well as definite moral codes. It was a mother's job to make sure all these intricacies of behavior were known and followed, especially by daughters, who stood the most to lose if they didn't stay within the lines. We needed Mother to teach and protect us, but at the same time we chafed under the load.

She became, perhaps beyond her wishes, the enforcer of society's rules and values, identified in my mind with them. She wanted what was best for us, but what was best was defined by what society had in mind. She operated to a large extent out of fear, anxious that Betty or I might go off the track. Perhaps she knew how cruel the ubiquitous, all-powerful "they" could be.

If you see your mother as the enforcer of society's values, and if you define yourself (as so many women of my generation did) in opposition to those values, then it's hard to become the mother. At least that was true in my case. So maybe in a way I took my youthful rebellion too far, refusing unconsciously all those years to become a mother because that was what my own mother wanted me to do, as if becoming a mother were the ultimate form of being "nice."

But like everything else, it wasn't that simple. For one thing, the times they were a'changing. Assassinations, drugs and rock, the sexual revolution, the women's movement, Vietnam: the world she had been grooming me for was disappearing right before my eyes. For so many of my generation, becoming our parents no longer seemed an option. And in that era when everything turned upside down, even if we didn't always know who we were, at least we knew who we weren't: our mothers and fathers.

Until we discovered, that is, that they were there in us all along. I felt that my current interest in becoming a mother had a lot to do with my own mother. At some level I wanted to get back to her. To become her, after all.

There wasn't a single word for what I felt for her. She was my mother, the most complex and probably the most important relationship of my life. She had carried me in her body, given birth to me, made sure I wore braces so my teeth would be straight, infuriated me when she criticized me, made me laugh with her sharp humor, been my best friend and most worthy adversary, made me do right, stood by me through everything, even when I wasn't sure I wanted her to.

Okay, I didn't really want to be that nurse— though it did have its appeal.

9

It had come to this: I was lying in bed, holding my hips up in the air so the sperm wouldn't run out on the sheets. We had made love this morning, and now I was trying to ensure that the sperm stayed in there, up there, long enough to make their wiggly way to the waiting egg. I had read that one reason women didn't get pregnant was that they leapt out of bed too soon after intercourse. The trick was to lie there for about fifteen minutes with your hips up in the air. But my arms were getting tired and I wanted to let go. Maybe if I couldn't hold my hips up in the air for a few minutes, I wasn't really mother material.

I directed my attention internally, to see if anything had taken in there. I pictured a skinny tadpole sperm caroming into a big fat (old) egg. What a shock it would be, a head-on collision. I saw the egg, blue as a planet, sticky like the lens of an eye. To tell the truth, I couldn't really imagine another being taking up residence inside me. It reminded me of what my mother taught me to call over the stall of the ladies' bathroom whenever someone else tried to get in: "Excuse me. Occupied. There's already someone in here."

I heard Jeff shaving in the bathroom, mindlessly singing a song from Ry Cooder's *Bop till You Drop* album: "Little sister, won't you please, please, please." I pictured him swaying in front of the mirror, mouthing the words as if he were a real soul man instead of a thirty-seven-year-old WASP lawyer. He used to dance naked to that record in front of the dark picture window of our apartment in Washington State, when he was in law school. Thank goodness the window faced onto a grove of Douglas fir. I remembered sitting on the couch, laughing and wondering, wondering and laughing. It didn't seem possible that someone who could dance the funky chicken naked, his big hands waving like a hula dancer's, could be going off to classes in contracts and civil procedure in the morning.

How had I managed to marry this person, who made me laugh and actually pleased not only me but my mother. It took my breath away. When I thought back to our beginnings, it seemed so hit-and-miss, so capricious, really, that we had gotten together.

After Pete I thought I had learned my lesson. I told myself I would not fall in love again with the wrong man. I'd fall in love with the right man. I'd make sure.

In the meantime a couple of men fell in love with me, or wanted to, if I would let them. I would not. I wasn't available. But then a man named

Wilson, someone I had known in the past, in California, before I got involved with Pete, contacted me again. He was in graduate school at the University of Chicago and he wanted to see me. He flew to Minneapolis.

Surely Wilson was the right man. He was certainly a nice man. I tallied up his attributes: a lovely small face, darling in its masculine way; an almost completed Ph.D.; intelligence; sensitivity; support for who I was and what I wanted to do. And he loved me. It didn't make sense that such a perfect man loved me, but he did. I could see that given a little time, things would lead to marriage. I was afraid of marriage, afraid of wanting it, afraid of not getting it. But maybe with the right man, the perfect man, maybe with Wilson it would work out.

It was during this same spring that I had this rather offbeat student from St. Paul named Jeff in my advanced fiction-writing class. He was taking graduate courses in the business school, toying with the idea of an M.B.A., but some internal divining rod had pulled him over to the creative-writing department.

People had to submit writing samples to get in the class, and I had found Jeff's manila envelope under my office door one day. It was a journal he had written when he had driven alone to California after graduating from college. There was something so lyrical in the prose that I pictured an awkward, sensitive guy. I figured he'd be the silent type in class, someone I'd have to draw out, so I was not prepared for Jeff in person. He wore baggy khaki pants and a plaid lumberjack shirt, and looked robust at the end of March in his big winter boots and overcoat. There was something appealingly masculine about him, and he had beautiful manners. But there was something oddball about him, too. I found myself looking to him in class for the astute comment, but sometimes the comment was not so much astute as irreverent or off the wall. And he would be laughing inside, I could see that, and for some reason I would be laughing, too.

Many of the students in that class were in graduate school, or adults from the community, older than me. We would all go to drink beer together after class at the Vali, a pizza parlor down some steep dark stairs in Dinkytown near the U. One day toward the end of the school year, I looked across the beer-stained table we were all crowded around and noticed a little puff of dark hair exploding at the base of Jeff's throat, just above his plaid cotton shirt. A wave of desire passed over me. I got to my feet, excused myself, and went to the bathroom. I sat in a stall with my face in my hands. No, I couldn't be doing it, it couldn't be happening. I was planning to go to Chicago for the summer to live with Wilson. Wilson was clearly the right man for me, the perfect man, and Jeff was clearly neither right nor perfect. He was, in fact, something of an enigma. He stayed on the periphery of our group, like a skittish dog, as if he wanted to join, but didn't know how. The story he had written for class was called "The Loneliest Man in the World."

I drove down to Chicago in June with Cecil and Creepy in my Volkswagen camper. Wilson liked the cats, he wanted to make friends. They, of course, wanted nothing to do with him, but we did all manage to live together. Only, what was this? My mind was straying back to Minneapolis, to a certain off-beat student in business who had taken my spring quarter class. Why should I, if I were honest with myself, admit that I couldn't wait for fall to come, so that I could see him again? I was screwing up! I must put him out of my mind. Clearly it was a perverse mind. Still, I got that same flush of desire when I remembered how the dark hair poked out of his plaid shirt at the base of his throat. The more I tried to put this image out of my mind, the more it popped up. All right. I would do this one thing: I'd send Jeff a postcard, no harm in that, perfectly normal, innocent, casual, we were friends after all, and I wouldn't even put my return address, I wouldn't even sign my name, too formal or something, I'd just sign it—P.

Summer came to an end, and now I was the bad person. The wrong person. The person who said she'd love and then couldn't, didn't. I left Wilson and drove back to Minneapolis with the cats. When I crossed the St. Croix River, which I knew Jeff sailed on sometimes, I felt like shouting with joy.

·

Finally I called him. I wanted to let him know that I was back in town. Did you get my postcard, I asked him. Oh, he said slowly. I wondered who "P" was.

It was rough sledding. Something was off in Jeff, at least in my opinion. He was odd. He liked me, it seemed, but he never made a move. It didn't come up, so to speak. Nothing was ever said, nothing was done. We acted as if we were friends. We *were* friends. But I was waiting, and nothing was happening.

Finally I decided I had to take some action. I invited Jeff to go up to the North Shore for a weekend to see the leaves. That ought to give him the hint!

It didn't.

We slept in separate rooms in a Grand Marais hotel. Later when we talked about it he explained that he thought I really wanted to look at leaves. Later still he said that he had thought I was still involved with Wilson. Later yet: "I didn't want to risk losing you as a friend."

Finally one night at a restaurant, I told him straight out. He made us leave the restaurant before I had finished my dinner. Now that he knew, he couldn't wait. He pulled me through the door of my place, and cats ran everywhere.

The next thing I knew, I was on my way to Tacoma, Washington, to live with Jeff while he went to law school. Almost a year had passed, but things were still not that certain between us. He wasn't sure. At least he wasn't sure he was sure. As for me? I was sure I wanted to try. That was as far as I was willing to go, in addition to Tacoma.

We drove our cars in tandem, his Mustang and my old V.W. bus, full once again of plants and cats. We traded off, since my radio had stopped working long ago. As we were crossing the Rockies, and Jeff was driving my bus, Creepy rubbed up against his leg, and he sneezed. He kept on sneezing. Thus we discovered Jeff was allergic to cats.

There we were, on the edge of the continent, two strangers practically, and he was allergic to cats. We checked into a motel until we could get our bearings, find a place to live. We didn't know a soul in town, and he was facing law school in two weeks, a terrifying prospect. I had left my job at the university. It wasn't as if I were quitting a tenure-track position. I had gotten some writing done the two years I was there, but I thought maybe I'd get more done away from full-time teaching. And besides, I figured that if I didn't go to Tacoma, that would be it for Jeff and me.

It was a difficult time. Tacoma, it turned out, was not a wonderful place to be. It was a strange, alien landscape to us. The law school was in a business park, a nondescript building that had a certain aggressive anonymity, a look of the little person struggling to pull himself up in the world. It was not a prestigious law school, but a law school for people who couldn't get into prestigious ones. Jeff had always thought of himself as special, but the law school shouted that he was not special at all, that he was one of many, and he'd be lucky if he were still enrolled a year from now.

It was raining and raining all the time, and Jeff was so disoriented, so topsy-turvy, that he left his good new Burberry somewhere, and we could never find it. We were frantic to find a place to live, to get out of the motel, to have some semblance of normalcy before Jeff began law school. I could tell how much it meant to him, how it was, in some way, a desperate gamble.

Jeff's was not a simple story where law school was concerned. He had suffered a grave head injury in an automobile accident when he was eighteen that had almost killed him. He had gone on to Princeton the next fall, but had had to drop out after the second year until the right combination of medications could be found to control his petit mal seizures. He still took Tegretol for what he called "spells," episodes lasting a few seconds in which he'd get a strange, déjà vu feeling from the scar tissue on his brain.

At Princeton his major had been English, for what he liked best was reading and writing. But the job market for English professors wasn't great. He came from a family of high achievers; his father and both brothers were surgeons. Jeff felt he had to prove himself, make something of himself. Being a lawyer was finally the thing he had come up with, but with some reluctance, some sense of biting the bullet.

There was something very dreamy about Jeff, something very funny, very fine. Law school was none of these things, but how do you turn being dreamy and funny and fine into a living? Not only a living, but a good living, as certain parts of his life demanded. Certain parts of himself. It was a desperate time, really, that time in life when important things were being decided—but for the people involved, the questions of the moment obscured, thank goodness, the monumental significance of it all: where shall we eat tonight, where are we going to live, where did I leave my damn raincoat, should I buy another? And what should we do about the cats?

I said I'd have them put to sleep. "That's the only solution, as I see it," I said. "We'd never find a home for two such scaredy-cats. My parents can't take them. You can't live with them. There's nothing else we can do." I was trying to be strong, but I felt like something was dying inside.

We were in his Mustang, with the want ads, looking for an apartment for rent, and it was raining. We had been driving around in the rain for days, looking for a place to live. We had left Cecil and Creepy back at the motel, which didn't allow pets. I was afraid a maid would come in to clean and they'd escape. At night we snuck them into my Volkswagen camper so Jeff wouldn't sneeze all night.

"We need to think about it," Jeff said. "Not make a bad decision." He glanced over at me. "I like Cecil and Creepy. I don't want to think of putting them to

sleep. And I'm afraid of what that would do to you."
Then after a moment he added, "To us."

I nodded. On the surface we got along well. We
were both reasonable, considerate, kind people. But
on another level, I felt we hardly knew each other.
We had been lovers for a year, and we were still cir-
cling one another, both too wary to get very close.
But at the deepest level, I did know Jeff, I knew
everything about him I needed to know.

"Here's something," I said, looking at the want
ads. "A 2 BR apartment for rent at a complex called
'Chateau in the Trees.'"

"'Chateau in the Trees?'" Jeff repeated incredu-
lously. We raised our eyebrows at each other, but
we were too tired, scared, demoralized, and damp
to laugh.

Chateau in the Trees was a newer complex with
cedar-sided units. Soldiers from Fort Lewis were
washing their cars in the parking lot to loud music
on their car radios. There were plastic squirrels on
the trees around the office and a tennis court out
back. In the distance we could see Mount Rainier.

"There are a lot of trees," I said carefully. The
complex was right on the edge of a forest of Douglas
fir. It was the sort of place I had never imagined living in in my life, a place where anonymous people
lived, not people like Jeff and me.

"It's close enough to the law school for me to get
there in about ten minutes," Jeff said hesitantly. "And
yet not too close." He looked pale, strained, and I
wondered what would happen. I wondered if he

would even go to law school, let alone make it through. There was a big battle going on inside him, over what he felt he had to do versus what he preferred not to do.

The office manager showed us an apartment on the second floor, with a combined living room/dining room and two empty bedrooms with brown carpeting and white walls. I couldn't imagine how we'd ever make a home of it. We could live there but it would always be a rental apartment that had nothing, ultimately, to do with us.

But it did have a little balcony out from the living room that was so close to the green fingers of the Douglas fir that I could reach out my own fingers to touch them.

Jeff joined me on the balcony. We leaned on the railing, breathing in the deep fragrant forest. We were both a long way from home. All we had was each other.

"I'm sorry I dragged you out here," Jeff said. "You don't have to stay, you know."

We were both silent for a long time.

"You didn't drag me out here," I said. After a while I added, "I wanted to come."

We were silent for some time. I couldn't tell which way things would go.

"We can keep them on the balcony!" Jeff suddenly exclaimed.

I looked at him in surprise.

"It's mild here all year, not like in Minnesota! Cecil and Creepy can live out here!"

I stared at him. Then I started laughing, out of joy.

"They'd love it out here," Jeff was saying glee-fully. "And you can come out and visit them, and they can come in sometimes. You see, don't you?"

I did see. And as we regarded each other on that dripping balcony at Chateau in the Trees, I saw a lot more.

Jeff started law school, and he had a hard time catching on.

"I was an English major," he'd exclaim. "I'm used to a lot of bull. I was so good at it at Princeton. But it doesn't seem to work with law."

One day I came in from getting some groceries to find him sitting on a bar stool in the dark apart-ment.

"What's wrong?" I rushed over to him.

He shook his head. "It's just so much," he said, and his voice broke. His shoulders shook. "It's just *too* much."

I had never seen him cry. It frightened me.

"It doesn't matter," I said. "If you can't do it, you'll do something else." But I knew that this might be it for Jeff. He had staked a lot on law school.

He sighed deeply. I put my arms around his back, which was slouched over. I held him tight.

"I'll fix you some supper," I said. "You'll feel bet-ter after you eat."

"Then I'll have to get back to the books," he sighed. "I have a midterm in civil procedure tomorrow."

Every night he'd study in the extra bedroom, trying to absorb endless case histories, sets of facts, rules of law. Every day he'd go off to classes. At night he'd grind his teeth in his sleep. I was alone a lot, and lonely.

I got a job as a waitress at a restaurant called "Poseidon by the Sea."

Poseidon by the Sea was a big Victorian house on the Sound; we had to wear long skirts and ruffled white blouses, as if we were in a play. The owners were ignorant retired army people who treated the waitresses as servants. The "chef," as he insisted on being called, was a retired army fry cook, a bully who would mess up or delay your orders if you didn't laugh at his sexist, racist jokes. I wasn't a particularly good waitress. I'd get flustered if the restaurant was too busy, forgetting which customer wanted extra blue cheese dressing and who needed more napkins.

I lasted about three months. Then I got a job as a teaching assistant at the school attached to the state institution for the mentally retarded, working with a class of severely retarded teenagers. After several months with this class, I was transferred to another classroom of less retarded, educable children who were severely physically handicapped.

I was writing short stories, though I was exhausted from my job a lot of the time. I was finding out what a lot of other people have found out, that making a living can kill off a writer.

After Rainier School I worked for the Department of Developmental Disabilities, on a CETA job, helping parents secure services such as respite care and equipment so they could keep their children at home.

When funding for that job ran out, I moved to another CETA job at an organization that educated the public about child abuse and neglect. I wrote scripts for a group of actors who would perform humorous skits containing parenting information in such places as the welfare office, the mall, and at the women's prison. I liked my job so much that we stayed on in Tacoma for a year after Jeff finished law school so that I could continue it.

After the first hard year of law school, Jeff had caught on. When he graduated, he got a job clerking in the state attorney general's office, defending cases brought by parents of handicapped children who wanted more than the state was willing to provide in terms of "mainstream" public education—or, as Jeff put it, "basically trying to deny the handicapped their rights under the law."

By then we had been in Tacoma for four years, and the question was, should we stay in Washington, or should we move back to Minnesota? And what about marriage?

We were trudging up a hill in old Tacoma. We had moved to the top of a duplex there from Chateau in the Trees. There was a big three-season porch where we kept the cats.

"I think we should move back to Minnesota," Jeff was saying. "My family is there, you liked it there, we both have friends there. There really isn't much to keep us here."

That was true. We weren't really "living" in Tacoma. We were just there on an extended visit.

"And I think if we move back, we should get married."

"But I already feel married to you," I hedged. "Why not go on happily the way we are?"

"Marriage is different," Jeff said. "It's different from just living together."

That was what I was afraid of. But secretly I was excited. I was ready to get married, too, only I couldn't quite bring myself to it without some coaxing.

It was 1980. I was thirty-three years old. I wouldn't have been able to get married in the seventies, I realized. For me the seventies had been about not getting married. I had spent the decade since college trying *not* to get married.

But now I had lived with Jeff for four years. I loved him. Marriage—at least marriage with Jeff—wasn't threatening to me anymore.

"Let's do it," I said.

"Okay," Jeff said. "We'll get married."

We had reached the top of the hill. Below us Puget Sound was spread out like a blue quilt.

I suddenly put my hand on his arm. "But how?" I said. "Do we have to have a wedding and all?"

"That's usually the way people do it," Jeff said.

"The only thing I know about weddings is that your mama takes over. I can't see myself at age thirty-three in a white wedding dress going down an aisle to be given away by my father."

"We're supposed to go to the bride's hometown to do it."

"Going back to Greenville to get married! That would be like saying uncle. It'd be like my mother won out, after all. And think of the expense! My parents couldn't afford it. I wouldn't even want to put them in that position."

"We could just do it here, in the courthouse," Jeff said. "Of course our families might be disappointed."

"Or mad," I said. "After all, getting married isn't a private affair. It signifies that you're joining society. You're going to fit in, after all." I suddenly felt very skeptical and suspicious of the whole thing.

"So what do you have in mind?"

"Nothing," I said. "I know exactly what I don't want in the way of a wedding, but I have no idea what I do want."

We finally decided to get married in Tacoma, in a small ceremony at the courthouse. I wanted to downplay the whole thing, because the idea of actually marrying was so momentous to me. Also, it seemed more "adult" to do it that way, on our own. I wanted to act adult because at some level I still didn't feel very adult. Adulthood was a fluctuating state.

Even planning for such a minimalist wedding still seemed to me to involve innumerable details

and decisions. When Jeff announced to his folks that
we were getting married, his father had asked what
we were going to do about a ring. Neither of us had
thought about a ring. I knew I didn't want a dia-
mond and band, but did I want any ring? And if so,
what kind? I was beginning to see the advantages of
letting your mother take over.

We decided to have a ring made by a goldsmith
in Seattle. On that May day in 1980 when we went
to pick it up, all the cars on I-95 between Tacoma
and Seattle were pulled off on the shoulder. We
pulled over, too. In the distance a huge mushroom
cloud, like the pictures of mushroom clouds after
atomic bomb explosions, dominated the sky. But this
was no atomic blast. Mount St. Helens had erupted.

Volcanoes were erupting and I was getting married. I wasn't sure which was the stranger phenome-
non. Now that we were going to do it, I was actually
quite happy about it. I had resisted the institution
of marriage with such a vengeance because I was
secretly deeply attracted to it.

"You'll want to register," my mother said as we
talked over some of the endless details on long
distance.

"Register for what?" I almost blurted out. Then
I remembered. "But I don't want any gifts, really," I
said. "I mean, we have everything we need, really."

"I'll sign you up here in Greenville," my mother
said. "My friends will want to give you something,
and it's a courtesy to give them some idea of what
you want."

My mother picked out a china pattern for me, something I would never have chosen on my own, and which I eventually exchanged for something I did like. She signed me up for pewter goblets and place mats. Despite my efforts to remain nonmaterialistic as part of my generation's antibourgeois rebellion, I began to look forward to the UPS truck bearing wedding gifts such as silver trays, steak knives, mixing bowls, crystal vases.

I didn't know what to wear to the wedding. Jeff could just wear a dark suit, but what could I wear? I didn't own any dressy dresses; I had given up such clothes along with panty girdles, French Provincial furniture, and Bill Nelson. But I did want something special for the occasion. I went to Saks in Seattle and paid too much for a maroon silk shirtwaist dress with tiny fleur-de-lis all over it, like a man's tie. It was an extremely conservative dress, something a woman would wear to a board meeting, not at all anything I'd normally wear. I didn't know what you wore to your wedding if you were a thirty-three-year-old nonvirgin feminist who had been living with someone for four years.

Finally the day came. We had been so low-key about the whole thing that I expected to be very cool and calm. But right before we left for the courthouse, I had a sudden attack of diarrhea. My bowels just let go. I could hardly believe my body. But it had its own truth: I was about to take one of the biggest steps of my life.

Our next-door neighbors, whom we liked but

hardly knew, met us at the courthouse to be our witnesses. Two friends of mine from work were there, and one of them took photographs. The judge, whom we had never met, wore a plaid green sports coat and looked like Milton Berle. He read from a sheet of standard wedding vows that we had approved beforehand. When he asked us to repeat the vows, Jeff was moved to tears. My own voice was strong and sure.

After the wedding we went back to our neighbors', who had a little reception for us. There was a three-tiered wedding cake, and they insisted on saving the top layer for me, to put in the freezer to eat on our first wedding anniversary. Saving the cake top was more important to them than to me. Jeff and I were about the least sentimental people I knew. We were full of sentiment, I felt—deep feeling—but we weren't very sentimental. I took the cake home and froze it, but I'm not sure what happened to it when we moved back to Minneapolis at the end of the summer.

For our honeymoon we drove to Seattle and spent two nights at the Olympic Hotel. That was all the wedding and honeymoon I could take.

But a wedding is only the barest beginning of a marriage. It is not marriage itself, which happens slowly over time, invisibly, incrementally.

10

In May we flew out to California to spend my fortieth birthday with Lauren and Allen. We went to Yosemite, along with Sarah Wilson, who was a friend of Lauren's and mine; we had all been in a women's group together in the seventies. Now they were both forty-one and I was turning forty. None of us had had children. We had all married in our thirties, and now Sarah was divorced. I missed the children my friends might have had. Lauren and I were trying to get pregnant, and Sarah had wanted a child while she was married, but now it seemed unlikely she'd have one.

It wasn't that we had postponed childbearing. I couldn't recall us ever discussing it back in our twenties. Maybe we had assumed, without even thinking about it, that we'd always have the possibility, out there sometime in the future, of children. But we were so busy back then with our own lives that we didn't miss or long for them.

My friends and I had had choices beyond anything our mothers had known. But those choices had had costs and consequences. Now, in our early forties, we were taking stock, considering the trade-offs. We had started off with such a sense of endless possibilities. And we had become, in so many ways, the women we had envisioned, the women we wanted to be. I looked upon my friends with great pride and joy; they really were terrific people. But I also saw that we all had given up certain things in order to gain others, often without realizing it.

Being with my friends, feeling not so much an age, a number, as just myself, I found that I was not ready to give up on having a child. I was finally at a point where I deeply desired one. It was funny, but now that I had turned forty, I felt readier to take it on. I was at the beginning of a new decade, and I felt like a young forty, not an old thirty. And I also knew it was now or never. Maybe we could still slip under the wire. A lot of older women, women just like me, were getting pregnant and having babies. Perhaps it would still work out.

When we got back from California, I made an appointment with my gynecologist to begin fertility testing.

Patty Hart, my gynecologist at Women's Health Care Center, was the kind of serious, bright girl all the other girls liked in high school, but whom the boys considered only as a pal. At my initial meeting with her I was full of worries and concern about what I was embarking on, wringing my hands, fretting. I hadn't wanted to have to arrive at this moment, where I had to be talking about possible fer-

tility problems. But Patty was straightforward, out-
lining what steps we'd take to investigate whether
something was wrong or not. We'd start with the
simplest, least invasive procedures, she explained.
There was something reassuring in the order that
she imposed on the situation, the idea that there
was a definite path to tread, and she'd take me by
the hand. When I left the office, I was excited and
relieved. I had finally begun fertility testing, as I
thought of it, but what I didn't know was that I was
still in kindergarten.

The first thing she did was have Jeff's sperm
checked out. He got back an excellent report, all
systems go, so we moved on to me, to a Huhner test.
Jeff and I had intercourse one morning, and then I
went in so Patty could extract some of the mucus to
see if the sperm were alive and well. From between
my upraised knees, she held up a two-pronged
instrument with a silvery string of my mucus suspended from prong to prong. "Fantastic," she said.
"Spin. You have great mucus."

I doubted that anyone else would ever say that
to me. I felt the warm glow of accomplishment and
was reminded that I would accept strokes for just
about anything.

I joined Patty at the microscope, where she was
observing the interaction of the sperm with the
mucus. "Want to see?" she asked, and I was brought
back to my high school days, the last time I looked
through a microscope. I bent my head, adjusted the

eyepiece and focus, and Jeff's sperm came into view, exactly the way I'd seen them in films about reproduction, only now I was looking at *Jeff's* sperm, wiggling around in *my* mucus. It was black and white, like an old movie, and other wiggles made their way across the field, strange strings of who-knew-what. "This is amazing!" I exclaimed, and a nurse-midwife passing by laughed. I felt deeply excited and interested, and expansively fertile. It had taken me a long time to arrive at this moment.

The mucus and my temperature chart indicated that I was near ovulation, and Patty sent me home with some Ovusticks, amazing little strips to stick in my urine to see if I was having an LH surge. New words were entering my vocabulary at a rapid rate now. Lutenizing hormone, which I had never heard of before in my life, was what activated ovulation. The stick turned a bright blue—an LH surge for sure—which meant I would ovulate in twenty-four to forty-eight hours. The egg would only be viable for twelve to twenty-four hours, so timing was essential. That night we made love, telling each other how much we loved each other, how wonderful it would be to have a child. I didn't see why it wouldn't work. In the morning my temperature had risen five-tenths of a degree, indicating ovulation had occurred. I lay in bed for a while, wondering if I were pregnant, if only by a few hours. It was hard for me to believe I wouldn't conceive, now that we were involving outside help. But I also knew that the chances of actually getting pregnant were small, only 10–15 percent on any given cycle Patty had told me, if everything goes perfectly. I didn't want to get my hopes up too much. I looked over my old temperature charts, and saw that we had actually hit my fertile period a number of times, as well as missing it completely. Still, it might work. People did have babies, it occurred to me. I might be one of them.

At work Jeff was embroiled in a difficult case, involving fraud in the sale of a furniture business. It all turned on accounting, and Jeff didn't know much about accounting. He had an accountant as an expert witness to help him with the financial statements, but he had trouble understanding him. "It's like this," Jeff tried to explain to me. "The accountant says two plus two equals four, and I go, 'Now let me get this straight. Two plus two equals four? Is that four, like four? I mean, do you mean an actual four? Could you show me with these pencils?'" We were both laughing, but every night Jeff was taking Valium to get some sleep.

Patty had scheduled me for a series of blood tests during the second half of my cycle, to see if my endometrium—another new word—was able to sustain a pregnancy. When I went in to have my blood drawn, I realized that I was happier than I had been in a long time. My fears and doubts hadn't gone away exactly, but they had receded in importance. I found myself fantasizing about having a child. Who would the person be who would come from Jeff and me? I felt a sense of amazement that Jeff and I might actually produce another person, out of our own two bodies. If it happens, Jeff said, it will be a miracle. He wasn't a religious person, but he couldn't help but talk about it in religious terms: It will be as if God waited on us.

I was waiting to see if I would start my period. I knew I probably would, but what if I didn't! I gave in one afternoon to reading about having a baby. I let myself go, something I had never done before, looking at pictures in a book a friend had lent me called *A New Life*, of a woman actually giving birth, reading her words about how she felt, and wondering all the time if I could be pregnant. My breasts felt slightly swollen and tender, which I thought might be an early sign—it was still a week until my period was due—and I noticed I was tired by the afternoon, but that might be from getting in three hours of writing before noon.

One morning my temperature dropped below ninety-eight. I called to make an appointment with Patty, since I was supposed to come in during my next period. I started my period that night. I had no idea why conception hadn't occurred. I felt disappointed, and a little mystified. But I didn't let myself get too down. There was still time.

When I went in to see Patty I got a shock. The blood work showed I had low progesterone, she told me—a 9. The scale was 2.5–28.1, so I was "normal," but they'd like to see at least a 15 to sustain a pregnancy. I needed to have an endometrial biopsy, in which a little bit of the lining of my uterus would be scraped off at a certain point in my cycle to see if it were rich and thick enough after ovulation. If it wasn't, that would confirm a luteal phase defect.

I had suddenly matriculated into first grade. I wandered out of her office in a daze. Something was actually wrong with me. I had a luteal phase defect, which sounded as if something were off with the moon instead of my hormones. When I got home I called Jeff. "I love you so much it doesn't matter if we have a child or not," he said, but I still felt as if I'd blown a fuse.

I looked up *luteal phase defect* in one of the books I had bought. Perhaps 3–10 percent of women have luteal phase defect related to hormone deficiencies, I read. It was more likely to be found in adolescent women, postpartum or perimenopausal women, and women over the age of thirty-five. It was sometimes treated, as Patty had told me, with Clomid, a drug that told the brain to make more estrogen. Clomid was the drug Lauren was taking. When she had first told me she was going to take it, I thought, *A fertility drug! How extreme. I would never go that far.* Maybe nature was trying to tell me something. Maybe it *was* too late. I remembered an article I had read recently on a single woman over thirty-five who just had to have a child, and did so with artificial insemination. But there was a postscript to the article, that the child had turned out to have progressive spinal muscular atrophy. I didn't know whether this was a genetic error related to the mother's age or not, but I was well aware that chromosomal irregularities could increase with age. I wondered again if maybe the wisest course wouldn't be to accept that the time had passed. When Patty had mentioned Clomid, she had talked as if it were no big deal. But I thought taking something like that into one's body, messing with one's hormones, was serious business. To me it meant another decision, and as usual I didn't know everything I'd like to know—such as, *Is this a good idea or not?*

"I hope it is low progesterone," Jeff said, "because then we'll know what's wrong, why you haven't gotten pregnant, and maybe it can be treated. Maybe it will turn out to be a simple problem with a simple solution." I could see what he meant, but I felt quite anxious over the whole matter. It made me feel so vulnerable: having something wrong with me, waiting for a test that I was frightened of (after all, she was going to *scrape my uterus*), taking a fertility drug, not to mention opening myself to the feelings I had had of hoping and even thinking I was pregnant.

When I went swimming one day at the Y, a woman was changing a baby on a blanket on the floor in the locker room. I watched them as I changed into my suit. I tried to see how I really felt about it. I didn't envy her, or see myself as wanting to be her—for one thing, the child looked so *big*. It was a lot of work and trouble to take care of a baby. Having a baby was one thing—but it was only one thing. Maybe it wasn't so sad not to have one. Maybe I was making too much out of it. Was there some way I could just close the door on it? I could see how that might be for the best.

I wasn't teaching during the summer, and every day I sat at my desk and wrote. I felt a constant worry over "producing" writing, which I figured contributed to my continuing stomach trouble. But at least I was hanging in there and writing. I unplugged the phone every morning, I got to bed on time, got up on time, got to my desk on time. I couldn't imagine that writing came harder for anyone. But I noticed that in spite of myself, I had become the person I had always wanted to be: someone sitting at her desk, writing.

I got my manuscript of short stories back from a university press contest, and to my surprise there was a letter informing me that I was one of ten finalists. I hadn't won the competition, but at least I had been a finalist. I was pretty thrilled. I seemed to know better and better what my book needed.

I went in for the endometrial biopsy, in which a little bit of the lining of my uterus was scraped off. This necessitated my cervix being held open with a tenaculum, a clawlike metal instrument of torture. I almost fainted when Patty did the actual scraping. She got a cold washcloth for my forehead, and I lay there for about fifteen minutes recovering from the pain. It had been much worse than I had expected. The pain had felt dark and primitive, primeval, uterine.

When the results were back in a few days, they showed that my endometrium was not working sufficiently to sustain a pregnancy. That was at least one possible reason why I hadn't gotten pregnant. (Could there be yet more reasons, more problems?) Patty said I could start Clomid after my next period, but I didn't know. I related my fears to her about forcing nature, that maybe my body didn't want to do this. She said not to worry about old eggs, because nature wouldn't let them "hatch." But I had read about Sally Quinn getting pregnant at forty and how the baby had a lot of problems. There were risks involved in trying to have a child at forty. Still, the thought of just ending—of not having some part of Jeff and me passed on—was very sad to me, almost unbearable at times.

September rolled around and I started a new school year. I had a kind of love-hate relationship with teaching. I hated how much of my time and energy it took, how tired it made me. But I also loved the students, most of them. I knew they were not the children I had never had, nor did I want to be their mother, god forbid. But I did feel a certain maternal attachment to them. I sometimes thought of how my mother had been a teacher before Betty and I were born, and I often felt the teacher in me was based on the teacher my mother had been. It was hard to separate mother and teacher. Actually, when I tried to think of a metaphor for how I felt as a teacher, what came to mind was a mother cat. It combined the maternal feelings I had for my students along with the fact that I also let them go. I'd see my former students around campus a year or two after they'd been in my class, and they'd be familiar to me, even dear, but I couldn't always recall their names. Over the years there had been so many litters, and there was always another litter on the way. While they were mine, I felt like I was doing the equivalent of nursing them (sometimes I felt they'd suck me dry), cleaning them up and teaching them what they needed to know. But I was always glad at the end of the term to see them go.

I called my father on his eighty-fourth birthday. His age was really beginning to show. If he went to the store, he couldn't remember what he was there for. But he always knew me when I called. I asked him what he wanted for his birthday. "Nothing!" he sang out. "Just for you to come home."

One day at the grocery store I saw the local quintuplets I had read about in the newspaper. There they were, five of them in strollers, causing quite a commotion. People who couldn't contain themselves over twins were having conniptions over the quints, cooing and chucking them under their five chins. The mother, I remembered reading, had been taking a fertility drug, Clomid, as I recalled. Taking

Clomid could result in multiple births. What would I do with two, three, four, *five* babies?

I started my period. I had known I would. And yet when I did, it was a blow. I had never expected to have to take a fertility drug. I wondered about the wisdom of it. But if I didn't take it, I would be giving up on having a child.

Now I said to Patty: Bring it on.

11

When I woke up on the Monday morning before Thanksgiving, I knew that this would be the day I would have Cecil put to sleep. Jeff had had to use his inhaler during the night, but then he was using it every night now, and I knew this was horrible, so horrible I couldn't go on living another day, doing him harm. I was crying. Jeff woke up and put his arms around me. "What is it?"

"I'm going to have Cecil put to sleep today."

We had known Jeff was allergic to my cats ever since that moment in my Volkswagen bus when we were driving to Tacoma and Creepy rubbed up against his leg and he started sneezing. But we had accommodated the situation over the years as best we could, mainly by keeping them in the basement. By now we had lost Creepy, who had died suddenly of a ruptured tumor. So at least we were down to one cat. We told ourselves that when Cecil died, we wouldn't get another cat. But Cecil seemed determined to stick around forever.

Over the past few years, in addition to his allergies, Jeff had developed asthma. Maybe he would have gotten it anyway. Or maybe, I thought horribly to myself, it was from living with a cat. And I determined to do the hard thing. Maybe we should get rid of Cecil, I'd say to Jeff every so often. And Jeff always talked me out of it. I like Cecil, he'd say. I don't think we should do it. And we'd drop it for a while.

But in October Jeff had caught a bad cold, and he had had trouble breathing. He'd decided he'd better see his doctor. He called me later that morning from his hospital room. The doctor had listened to his lungs and admitted him immediately, because of asthma.

I was alarmed and frightened. And guilty. Was I doing Jeff damage? Was I being a fool? I was, but that didn't seem to stop me. I couldn't seem to help myself.

Jeff spent several days in the hospital watching the Twins make it into the World Series. When he came home he had to use an inhaler often. "I could be allergic to anything," he said, for indeed he was allergic to all sorts of grasses and pollens. "I might still have hay fever if we got rid of Cecil," he soothed me, and the asthma, well, maybe he would have gotten that anyway, and at least it was under control.

But that Monday morning before Thanksgiving, I knew what I had to do. I was waking up around four every morning, guilty and troubled. I was up against something I couldn't deny or postpone any longer.

I knew that if I was ever going to be able to do it, I had to do it *now*, today. I wasn't strong enough to put it off, to try to find Cecil another home, which I knew would prove difficult, given his age and timidity. Any delay would give me time to equivocate, and then I wouldn't be able to give him up. If I was ever going to do it, I had to do it today.

Jeff had to help me. He had to do it, really. I had thought I could see it through, but I couldn't. We went to the vet's, my idea, to get a tranquilizer for Cecil. I would give it to him at home, and then he would be calm, sleepy, when he had to go to the vet's for the lethal injection. Cecil was always so frightened when he had to go to the vet's, and I didn't want him to be frightened. He had always been so afraid of everything, and I had promised myself that I would take care of him. Now that had to come to an end.

I gave him the pill, and Jeff went off to work. He would come home in a few hours to help me. I spent those hours with Cecil, holding him, stroking him, saying good-bye. Unfortunately the pill did not make him calm, it made him weird, not what I had had in mind at all. It made him terribly restless, his eyes dilated, and he seemed tortured by what I had put into his system. I tried to hold him, to calm him. Tears were streaming down my face.

Finally, when I thought I couldn't stand it another moment, Jeff came home. I had the cat cage ready, and I put Cecil inside. He looked out at me with his yellow dilated eyes. I had thought I could go to the vet's, I felt I should see it through, but I could not. Jeff, his face a mask of trouble, picked up the cage. He carried Cecil out. I ran to the window and watched them go. I followed the car in my mind all the way to the vet's. And still it was not too late. I could get on the phone, call the vet, tell them to stop.

But I didn't. I was finally doing what I should have done a long time ago, and I was glad for it. Sometimes it's necessary to sacrifice the very thing you love. I marveled, from inside a tremendous pain, that I could do it. I wouldn't have been able to, earlier. It had something to do with marriage. It had taken me a long time to become this deeply married.

When Jeff came home he looked ashen. "We don't have to make a pretense about talking about other things," he said. "Losing Cecil is what we want and need to talk about, and we can talk about it all we want."

We both missed Cecil terribly. I could see him everywhere, I could hear him coming up the stairs, the particular creak one of them made when he ran up to greet me in the mornings. But I was relieved he was gone. There were certain things that life demanded and a certain relief in facing up to them. And now, I thought deeply to myself, bargaining, maybe I'll be able to have a child. Maybe out of this loss, for reasons I can't fathom, a child will come.

When I called home on Sunday, I told Mama about Cecil, and she started crying on the phone. It was a great comfort to me to have her sympathy. My mother knew me, and she knew what it would mean to me to give up Cecil. I was glad Daddy wasn't home; he was so tenderhearted I couldn't imagine telling him myself. He would have been hurt to hear me hurt. They were my parents, and my pain was their pain.

I had invited Jeff's brother Peter and his wife, Mary Ellen, over for Thanksgiving dinner several weeks ago, and though Jeff and I were still suffering from losing Cecil, we decided to go ahead with it.

Peter and Mary Ellen had just had their first baby at the end of October. The birth of their baby, such a happy occasion for them, had brought me great pain. When we first heard of the birth, I cried as if my heart would break. Well: feeling sorry for myself. They had a baby, and I didn't, and I didn't know how to get one.

On our way over to the hospital to see the new baby the day after he was born, we had stopped and bought a tiny Twins World Championship T-shirt. The Twins had just won the World Series and had had a big ticker tape parade in downtown Minneapolis. Jeff had left his office to see it. If I ever have a child, he had said, I'll want to be able to tell him about it.

We found Mary Ellen's room on the sixth floor and there was a sign on the door, "Mother resting, no one admitted," under which was written in pencil, "unless your name is Jeff Alden." Jeff, very eager, opened the door, and Peter was lying on a bare cot, with Mary Ellen in the hospital bed. When Peter got up to greet us, I saw the bundle on the cot that was the baby. He had a head of dark hair, pursed lips, nicely shaped and rosy red, as if he had on lipstick, and a funny little chin that caused Peter and Mary Ellen to joke about how the baby had a weak chin. His eyes were shut the whole time we were there, and he had on white cotton mitts to keep him from scratching himself. John was a nice-looking baby, really big, they said, though to me he looked so little.

Seeing the baby, I felt somewhat removed from whatever it was that had broken my heart the day before. Faced with an actual infant, I felt uncertain. I didn't know how I'd feel if I knew from then on I'd be responsible for that child. It was nothing to take on lightly. I wanted a baby myself, but at the same time, I was afraid of it, and another part of me simply didn't want it. I did and I didn't.

Now they were coming over for Thanksgiving dinner with the baby. I cooked a big turkey and made dressing and gravy, and a yam dish called liquor pudding that we always had in South Carolina. Mary Ellen brought over the vegetable, salad, and pumpkin pie. After we were all stuffed we sat around in the living room, mostly looking at John. I would have liked to tell Peter and Mary Ellen about our infertility problems, about how I was in treatment, how we were trying to have a child, but there was never an opening to bring it up. At one point, when I was sitting next to Mary Ellen on the couch, she held the baby up and said, "We love him so much!" I had to get up and go in the kitchen by myself for a few moments then.

There was the pain of losing Cecil, and there was the pain of infertility, and sometimes they ran together and were the same. Pain was a peculiar thing. It made me feel strange; it made me retreat. I felt that my relationships to other people had changed in certain ways. I was carrying around a burden that only a few people knew about. It made me feel apart from most people, as if I could see them, but they were a long way away. People were going about their normal lives, and now I carried about with me all the time pain, as if pain were my child.

We decided to tell our families about our infertility treatment. It was such a big part of our lives now, and we felt alone and lonely about it. We wanted our parents' support, their advice, their understanding. It was hard to think of Christmas approaching, with its emphasis on family, children, and happiness. We felt things would be easier somehow if people knew what was going on with us. I wrote to my parents, and Jeff talked to his folks in St. Paul. It was a relief to me to have it out in the open. My mother called after they got the letter, and I poured out what it was like to be trying and not succeeding. I knew she would support my efforts to try to have a child, and now I needed that support.

Jeff's mother called me after their talk, and was very sympathetic. But at the end of the conversation, trying to spare me, she said, "We won't talk about this again. We won't mention it." I didn't know if that was what I wanted or not.

One day in early December I came home to find a letter from Graywolf Press, where my collection of short stories was under consideration. I sat on the radiator to warm up and read it. I skimmed the letter quickly, as I always did such letters, looking for the key words that would tell me whether the news was good or bad. In this way I attempted to protect myself from rejection. I was sure Graywolf would reject *Feeding the Eagles,* but I hoped they'd be kind about it, and maybe even throw in a compliment or two to ease the disappointment. It was the compliment I was searching for amidst the "sorry" part.

"I'm very sorry for our long delay in responding to your manuscript of short stories, Feeding the Eagles," the letter began. *"We put a great deal of effort into the books we publish, and feel a good deal of very personal commitment to them. We like to regard ourselves as publishers with heart, and sometimes it takes us time to come to allow ourselves to fall completely in love with a book."*

At least he had the decency to apologize for having had it for five months.

"We have, with yours, and if you are not utterly impatient with us for taking our time romancing your book, we would love to publish Feeding the Eagles.*"*

A strange tingling started at the top of my head. I felt as if I might levitate off the radiator. Graywolf was going to publish my book. *I was going to have a book.*

I called Jeff. I was stunned, amazed, in shock. Jeff began to make it real for me: "My wife the author!" he said joyfully. I called my writing pal Sasha. I called Lauren in California. Telling them made the news more real. I read the letter over and over. They wanted to publish *Feeding the Eagles* if I found this "a pleasant prospect." There was information about an advance, about royalty rates. They would be pleased, Scott Walker, the publisher, wrote, to help my work find readers.

Readers.

I waited a few days before I called my folks to tell them the news. I had never had to face the reality of publishing a book, and I needed a little time to get used to the idea. For one thing, what would my parents think? They were scattered all through the book. I had been writing the stories for years, and occasionally I'd published one of them in a small press journal somewhere, not exactly the sort of magazines my parents back in South Carolina kept up with. I'd been selective about what I'd shown them. Now I'd have to come clean. I was relieved that the publication date was a long way off. I needed time, and I knew my folks would need time too. I couldn't just spring the published book on them one day. I would have to show them the manuscript. I was glad I was so far away.

I could hear the tears of happiness in my father's voice when I told him the news. Anything that made me happy made him happy. My mother was thrilled too, but she immediately asked, "When can I read it?"

There was also the little matter of my sister. I had a story in the collection about her, and it wasn't all flattering. I thought it was loving, but that was different. Who was I to know how she would feel about it? How would I feel reading about myself through her eyes? That thought caused an uncomfortable feeling deep in the pit of my stomach.

I was waiting for my period again. Maybe now that I was going to have a book published, I would be able to have a child.

It was day twenty-seven of my cycle, and I felt crampy, full, as if I were going to start. But wasn't that a possible sign of pregnancy? My gynecologist, Patty, had said you might feel as if you were going to start and even bleed some, but you could still be pregnant. Of course it might be too early for my temperature to drop. I was starting my period later now that I was on the Clomid. I woke up off and on during the night, anticipating waking up at seven to take my temperature, wondering what it would reveal. If it had dropped, I'd know I wasn't pregnant. But if it hadn't, I'd still have a chance.

When I took it the next morning, it was still up there, 98.6, and I felt elated. I thought of waking Jeff to tell him that I was probably—*almost certainly!*—pregnant, but then I remembered how I had been suckered the previous month, and I didn't want to indulge in that kind of magical thinking again. Still, I got out of bed and went to check to see if I had actually started. I hadn't. Not yet.

I was scheduled for another endometrial biopsy, to see if the Clomid was having the desired effect on my endometrium. I was worried that the test might disturb a pregnancy if I had conceived, but it had to be done on day twenty-eight, and we decided to go ahead. It didn't hurt as bad as the other time. Since the last test Patty had discovered a new suction method that was quicker and less painful, and the results this time showed that the endometrium was thick and lush enough to sustain a pregnancy, good news.

The next test I would need was a hysterosalpingogram, which Patty had scheduled for a few days before Christmas, at a certain time in my cycle. When I first heard the word I could neither remember nor pronounce it, but after a few days I was slinging it around as if it were "boo." A hysterosalpingogram, commonly abbreviated as HSG, involved shooting dye through the fallopian tubes to see if they were open. The thought of this test caused me great anxiety; I felt queasy, weak in the knees, and what if the results were bad? What if the test showed my tubes were blocked, and had been all this time? Did I really want to know that? And if so, what then?

I really did seem to be missing my period. A few more days had passed, and my temperature was still up there, at 98.3, though it had dropped three-tenths of a degree, which I didn't know how to interpret. It was still over 98, and that was the important thing. I woke up sometime in the night too excited to sleep, thinking of my book and being pregnant. Could both be true?

At four I got up and stood at the window. Outside everything was hushed and still, and snow was falling in huge flakes, drifting down from the bright dark sky in lazy spirals. The garden was covered in a white blanket, as if deep asleep while I kept watch. I woke up again at six to take my temperature. I waited six minutes with the thermometer in my mouth. If down, no pregnancy. If up, *maybe*. It was up, by one-tenth of a degree.

I was sure I was pregnant. I just *felt* so pregnant. How could I not trust my own body, my own deep sense of what I knew to be true?

I told Jeff that I thought I was pregnant, and he told me I was acting nuts, setting myself up. I needed to wait a few days to see, he said.

The next morning my temperature was still up,

and I decided to go in for a pregnancy test. I had to know. If only I could get pregnant—that would at least mean that I could conceive. I couldn't even get to first base. Just getting pregnant seemed a major hurdle. That was all I was asking for right now. Just to be pregnant. *Please let me be pregnant.* Jeff was in suspense, too.

I took a sample of my urine into the clinic. Patty looked at my temperature chart. Too early to tell, she said. Take a deep breath and scream. Surround yourself with fertility objects. Do what women have done through the ages.

I needed to get home to work on a new course I was preparing, but I was too excited and preoccupied. I went to Hardee's for lunch, fretting that a fast food hamburger might be one of the baby's first meals. Afterward I went over to the Resolve office to read material on infertility and pregnancies. I had joined Resolve, a support organization for people experiencing infertility, and had been to one of their meetings. But I didn't identify with them too much. I was planning to get pregnant, so what would I need with an organization like Resolve?

When I called in to the clinic that afternoon, the urine test was negative. I was stunned. I had been so *sure.* But a blood test was much more accurate, they told me. I went back to the office to have my blood drawn, and settled down to wait until ten o'clock the next morning. An early urine test could be wrong, so I still had a fifty-fifty chance. What was I to do with this feeling, this certainty, that I was pregnant? How could I have that feeling, and not be pregnant? My breasts were swollen, I felt bloated and full, my temperature was still up there. I experienced every possible emotion in the next eighteen hours: the ecstasy of pregnancy; the agony of infertility; the miracle of a live birth; the pain of miscarriage; the tragedy of a stillborn; the uncertainties of a preemie or handicapped child; the joy of everything going great.

The next morning, my temperature was still right up there, 98.4. I was on day thirty-three of my cycle, and if I could just make it through this day without starting . . .

The blood test was negative. I couldn't believe it. I couldn't believe that I could be so fooled. So wrong. I felt vaguely humiliated, as if I'd made a fool of myself. Running with the ball before I caught it.

Jeff was looking around for office space. It was actually going to happen, he had actually given notice, he was quitting his job and going *solo*. The word made me feel as if the bottom were opening beneath us. I couldn't quite believe it was true, and he couldn't either. He told me about walking through the skyways at lunchtime and seeing all the bankers and lawyers in their suits and ties, and how he suddenly thought, *All these people are getting paychecks!*

He rented an office in the Lumber Exchange Building, to begin January 15. We went and ordered business stationery. We had both known that Jeff was unhappy in the firm, that it was only a matter of time before he'd leave. He wasn't looking into other firms, figuring he might very well be jumping from the frying pan into the fire. Going on his own suited Jeff, we both thought. But the reality of it all was still daunting.

The HSG was coming right up, and I was nervous on two fronts. I was worried that it might really hurt; the name, hysterosalpingogram, made me think of women hysterical with pain. And I was anxious about the results. "Women vary in their re- actions," they told me at the clinic, which I took to mean, *It can hurt like hell.* And what if my tubes were blocked? That felt like knowledge I'd just as soon avoid.

The day finally arrived, December 22, and I was sitting on the X-ray table in the examining room in my hospital gown, trying not to cry. I felt absolutely shaky with fear, as if I were going to whimper. Patty was late; I was always waiting for medical people. A small blond nurse told me what would happen. A catheter would be inserted into my uterus and then dye would be shot through my tubes, and if they were not blocked, things should go fine and they'd take photographs and that would be it. "I'm not going to lie to you," she said. "It can be very painful. Sometimes the tubes can go into spasms. And the test can take from five to ten minutes."

Finally Patty arrived in the X-ray room wearing a green surgical outfit. She and I had agreed that if I didn't get pregnant my next cycle, I should move on to an infertility expert. This thought made me sad, and I was sorry to have to leave Patty. I had been on Clomid five months, and at my age it would be better to be with a specialist who might escalate my treatment. I had made an appointment with a specialist for the end of January, the first I could get in, but I was hoping I'd never have to keep that meeting.

There were a few cramps when Patty inserted the catheter, but not too bad. Then almost before I knew it, it was over. The dye had run through smoothly, quickly, without a hitch. Everything looks great, Patty said. Your tubes are open. I was in shock. That was it? It was over?

Patty showed Jeff and me the films, which were fascinating to see. In one picture the white image of the dye spilled out of the left tube into a little galaxy-like configuration in the dark pelvic area. The other tube was partially hidden by the somewhat triangular uterus. It appeared twisted and shorter, but was perfectly normal, according to Patty. I stared at this inner landscape, trying to understand that it was me.

For Christmas we went over to Jeff's folks' house. The big news was that Jeff was going on his own, and of course the new baby, John, who slept through most of the festivities. I felt uncomfortable and awkward around the baby. I didn't really want to hold him. I felt self-conscious that we had told everyone that we were trying to have a baby. Maybe it would have been better if we had kept it to ourselves. By the end of the day I felt beaten down by the situation.

We stayed home on New Year's Eve, and as we were making love, I started to cry. It was losing Cecil, and it was my book being accepted for publication. It was my parents growing old, and it was thinking I was pregnant. It was the HSG and it was Jeff quitting his job. It was Peter and Mary Ellen's new baby, and it was the way sex was now connected to trying to conceive. It was all that, and more, things I couldn't even begin to name.

On that note, with me crying and us making love, we welcomed in the New Year.

12

In January I had lunch with Scott Walker from Graywolf. I felt shy and excited, but he was easy, accepting, and encouraging. He didn't say a lot about my book. "It's a quiet book," he said, "but that's what I like about it." Then he added that it wasn't going to sell to the movies.

Some nights I couldn't sleep because of visions of success swirling through my head. I dreamed of the book being favorably reviewed, being LOVED. On the other hand, what if it got panned or not reviewed at all? I expressed some of these fears to Scott, trying to keep my anxiety at an acceptable level. "It may do better than you expect," he said.

I had sent copies of my manuscript off to my parents and Betty, and I began to sweat it out. Of course, maybe it was a bit late in the day for me to be pretending I cared so much what my family thought. After all, the stories were a fait accompli. I had written them; several had been published. That caused me to brood about what sort of monster I really was. Maybe I really didn't care at all what my family thought. Maybe it was all for show, this pretense that I cared one iota for their feelings. But I did! I do! Yet I wrote the stories. I knew I wouldn't change them.

It was one thing, I was discovering, to write about your family, and quite another to publish that writing. But maybe my stories weren't really that bad; I wasn't in much of a position to judge. Still, they were full, it seemed to me, of family business. Private stuff. I wasn't really sure, myself, how revelatory they were. "Maybe they won't see it at all the way you do," my writing pal Sasha consoled me. "Maybe they'll be glad not to see themselves portrayed even worse."

That thought had never occurred to me.

I lay in bed with Jeff. He was reading; I was brooding. "I read that Annie Dillard let her family read her new memoir before she published it," I spoke into the air. "She said she'd let them censor anything that was in it." I shook my head. Maybe Annie Dillard was a much better person than I.

"If you let your family censor whatever you write," Jeff said, "you wouldn't write anything."

I told Scott Walker my fears. "Of course I don't know what my family is going to say about all this!" Brightly, as if I had it under control.

"It's a problem for almost everybody," he said calmly.

Finally the Sunday came when I had to call home (I called every Sunday). I figured my parents had gotten the manuscript on Thursday. I wasn't worried about my father. He wasn't a reader to begin with, and he was invariably uncritical where I was concerned, having the attitude since my birth that anything I did was fine with him. But my mother. Keeper of the rules, guardian of society's niceties. Her battle cry when we were growing up had been *"What will people think?"* which was maybe why I had written a book that would really give people something to talk about.

Finally the moment came. My mother and I had covered everything else we possibly could, and at last she said, "Well, I read your book, and I like some things about it, and I don't like some things about it."

I was reading a world in her voice. I knew that voice so well, every intonation, every pause, every inflection. I could tell I was probably home-free.

"Well, what did you like about it," I said, and I found I was grinning, out of happiness at finally confronting this moment.

"Well," my mother said, "I think you write with a lot of feeling. I found myself laughing and crying."

That didn't surprise me. It was, after all, the history of our family.

"What didn't you like about it?"

There was a significant pause. "The sex."

The sex, I thought. What sex?

"Ohhh, that!" I said finally. "The sexxxxxxx. Well, that part's all made up. That part's fiction!"

My mother laughed. I laughed. It was a nice moment.

Then we talked about the book. What amazed me was that none of the things I had worried about disturbed her. Or if they did, she didn't let on to me. When I asked her about the parts that I saw as particularly sticky, she said, "I think you told the truth." But what about *What will people think?* Actually, being my mother's daughter, I was plagued myself quite a bit by that question. I meant the people in Greenville, the people who knew my parents, my sister, me. If I had imagined an audience for the book, it was sophisticated, literate readers a few states away whom I would never meet, and not the women in my mother's bridge club.

"Well, maybe your publisher will send you down here for a reading," my mother said.

A reading? In my hometown? Showing my face in the light of day in Greenville, with that book in tow? I had to hand it to my mother. It occurred to me that maybe she was proud of me.

I had sent the book to my sister, Betty, in Virginia at the same time I had sent it to my parents. Days passed, weeks. No word. What did that mean? Did it mean she was angry? Was she offended? Hurt? I fantasized an angry letter in which she said she would never speak to me again. Or better yet—"If you publish that . . . that . . . *book*, I never want to see you again!" Then what would I do? It made me squirm to realize I didn't know.

My sister and I were so similar and so different. I felt more at home around her than anyone I knew, yet we often had different reactions to things. After her divorce she had gone back to school to get a Ph.D. in education and had embarked on an impressive career as school superintendent in several districts. In a lot of ways she was more liberated than I, a woman who had been burned by divorce and who had learned to take care of herself. Eventually she had remarried, to a man who had already raised two sons, and when she reached age forty, she had had her tubes tied, with very little expenditure of emotional energy. She was pragmatic, smart, dedicated to her work, and very into birdwatching.

Then one day a letter arrived. "Of course I got your book and I have been absorbing it," she began. "Reliving all the feelings, some of which I'd forgotten. I really don't remember a great deal about growing up, it's all sort of a blur. I found myself laughing and crying at the same time. I was drawn to the stories about or with me in them, but I also didn't want to know or be faced with myself through your eyes. I know there is a lot of truth in the beach story and that I don't necessarily like certain parts that are me, but I have to accept it. At any rate, I'm very pleased about the book."

I felt as if some huge weight had been lifted from my shoulders. My mother and sister—the two people I was most worried about—had passed on my book.

Jeff had called the Skywalker to meet him at his old office, and they moved his plants and pictures through the skyways of downtown Minneapolis to his new office in the Lumber Exchange. He had rented furniture, and had taken a few files. I went down to see him on his first day in the new office. He didn't even have a phone yet. The office was very nice, in an old historical building with beautiful woodwork and some of the original brick walls. There was a view out his window of Hennepin Avenue. It was all very exciting, but still there came the moment when we simply looked each other in the eye, taking stock. Now we'd be paying not only our house mortgage, but the rent on his office and all the expenses involved in running his own business. "I guess we'll eat what we kill," Jeff said.

We had our first appointment with Paul Kuneck, the infertility specialist at Abbott Northwestern Hospital. Dr. Kuneck had just opened the infertility clinic in August, and unlike the other infertility doctors in town, it didn't take six months to see him. He was about my age, with dark hair and a serious demeanor. He had been in private practice as a gynecologist before training as a specialist in infertility. He wore a white lab coat, and he seemed nice enough, though I noticed he related to me more than to Jeff. Perhaps he was more accustomed to women.

Jeff and I were full of questions. We asked him about our chances of having a handicapped child. The chances rise with age, he told us, but only to about 4–5 percent, as opposed to 2 percent in the general population. He didn't think it was ill-advised at my age to be pursuing pregnancy. Clomid didn't really force nature to do something it didn't want to do, and if the egg wasn't viable, it would abort. But the chances of miscarriage at my age were 25 percent or more, because of the eggs being old and genetically unviable. He said we really hadn't been trying all that long. He was full of statistics.

We scheduled another appointment for me for Friday, for another Huhner test, to see if the mucus was still conducive to the sperm, and I was going to have to have yet another endometrial biopsy, but not another HSG. Jeff felt after the meeting that we still had a good chance, and I felt the opposite. He saw the glass as half-full while I saw it as half-empty.

I had to have a pregnancy test before the endometrial biopsy, a precaution to make sure I wasn't pregnant, since the tube inserted into my uterus to suction a bit of the endometrium could disturb a pregnancy. No one in infertility treatment wants a pregnancy disturbed. I went in in the morning to have blood drawn, and by late afternoon I'd know. I didn't think I was pregnant. I had no expectations that I was. It was just a precaution, really, and had nothing to do with anyone thinking that I was pregnant.

At about three-thirty Linda from Dr. Kuneck's office called with the results. "Negative." *I'll say.* "That's what I expected," I said in a calm, bright, social voice. *It doesn't bother me!* I said I'd see her,

then, at half past eleven the next day for the endometrial biopsy.

I got into bed. I had a deep urge to be unconscious. I didn't want to be conscious for the next
hour of my life. I curled up under the covers, almost
crying, but I wouldn't let myself go. I didn't want to
give in to such an irrational pain. Still, disappointment poured over me. I was surprised to feel it
again, so acutely. And I had to face the biopsy the
next day.

It was interesting to go to Dr. Kuneck's office, because unlike the office of my gynecologist, I knew
what all the women were there for. They were all
experiencing some sort of infertility problem. They
all wanted a child they had not been able to have.
One day when I was there (for I was there a lot
now), a pink cyclamen arrived, and I immediately
exclaimed to Dr. Kuneck, who happened to be standing at the reception desk, Oh! Someone must have
had a baby. We haven't been here long enough for
anyone to have a baby, he said. But a patient had
had a positive pregnancy test. Someone had at least
made it that far. After that whenever I went in I saw
the cyclamen, still blooming beautifully. Pink. I kept
thinking of this other couple, Pam and Ray—I had
seen their names on the card—and I wondered if
she were still pregnant.

I was there for the endometrial biopsy, but I
needed to schedule future appointments. Linda, who

ran the office, was small and sweet and we were
getting to be friends. Today I needed to schedule an
appointment for the start of my period to see if
my ovaries were gigantic, a possible side effect of
Clomid. I also needed a conference to talk over the
latest blood test results, and the results of the endometrial biopsy. She couldn't find a day open when
I could do both at one time. That meant two trips to
the hospital next week. Then she said that Dr.
Kuneck probably wouldn't have time to read the
slide results by the following Friday, which upset
me. I didn't want to start Clomid again—the seventh
month of it—without knowing the biopsy results.
How could anyone with a full-time job manage infertility treatment? It was a full-time job itself.

I asked Linda how long the wait would be today.
There were three other women in the reception
room, and the last time I had been there, I had had
to wait forty-five minutes. I had gotten more and
more upset and angry, and strangely, I felt I would
cry. When I'd finally gotten in, I announced that we
had to discuss how long I had waited before we
could talk about anything else. Dr. Kuneck wasn't
defensive and was appropriately contrite. He said
he'd feel exactly as I did, which defused me, though
I still wanted to cry. Today I was prepared to wait
patiently and peacefully; I had brought along the
thickest book I could find, *Bonfire of the Vanities.*

Linda said the wait wouldn't be long, and in an
unbelievably few minutes Dr. Kuneck appeared and
called me into the examining room. He told me not

to stop taking my temperature after I ovulated, and I told him about the slide report problem. He said he would definitely read the results before I came in next Friday. I was beginning to like him. I hadn't disliked him before, it was just that he was so foreign to me, a little stiff and formal, and he always seemed burdened, serious. Maybe it was all those infertile couples on his mind.

I had taken a Motrin before the procedure, and since this was my third biopsy, I knew what to expect. I knew it would hurt but that I'd be able to stand it. While he was between my legs with the speculum, I leaned up to look at him, and said, "Can we talk or do you need your full concentration?" I was joking a little, but I didn't really know him well enough yet to know if he would want to talk while doing the biopsy. He was getting me ready, swabbing the cervix. He told me carefully what to expect. But what I wanted to ask was whether I'd be able to tell, before missing a period, if I were pregnant. That question haunted me every cycle, during the long stretch between ovulation and my period. He said no, most women can't tell at all. Though some women, he went on, had told him that they knew two days after getting pregnant. Their breasts felt more tender. Mine feel that way every cycle, I said. No, he said, it's different. Oh, different! I murmured. What would it feel like? I wanted to know, to feel it. The mysteries of a pregnant body seemed irresistible and unattainable to me.

He began the procedure. First he had to probe

to get the depth of the uterus. I began to hurt, to cramp deep inside, and then came the other sensation, the actual suctioning off of tissue from the uterus. It caused a deep, sickening pain, and it went on maybe fifteen seconds. I knew, because I was trying to endure it, and I kept having to ask, How much longer? How much longer! He said, about five more seconds, and I began counting, five, four, three, two . . . I expected him to keep his part of the bargain and get the hell out of there. It was over, and I lay there, still in pain, cramping, but beginning to feel better. That certainly is an unpleasant test, I said, and he acknowledged that it was. He said he always wondered what it might feel like, and the nearest he could come was having to go to the dentist. The dentist! I thought. Well, at least he was trying.

I felt extremely benevolent toward him afterward. He had hurt me all right, but not too much, and he had been kind, present. I thanked him, and I felt grateful that he understood that I needed to know about the slide results before the next round of Clomid. Still, those results would probably be only part of the puzzle, a piece of information in a larger conundrum. He told me my blood work was all normal except for what appeared to be an inverse ratio of the luteinizing and follicle-stimulating hormones, but that might be due to having the sample taken right at ovulation, and we'd check it out again. Tests, and more tests. My insurance company must have been going wild.

I lay on the examining table for a while after he left, rubbing my abdomen. But after a short time I got up and got dressed and went down to the coffee shop. It was twelve o'clock. I had arrived a little after eleven. I couldn't recall ever having a medical appointment go so speedily. Dr. Kuneck gained points for that. And I had an appetite! From pain to hunger—I was certainly restored to my old self. I felt rather fragile and in mild pain, but I ate a turkey sandwich, enjoying a few moments of solitude, the ordeal behind me. I contemplated my continuing state of nonpregnancy. The mind searches for something to latch on to. Well, maybe this was all for the best! Maybe I needed this test so we could know how things stood with my endometrium before I got pregnant. Things would be better that way, really. Then I thought about when I would have a child if I got pregnant: February, March, April, May, June, July, August, September, October. I counted up on my fingers. I might not teach fall quarter. Could I go back winter quarter? I'd want to. I bused my dishes and went out to find my car. It was one degree below zero.

13

It was time to make a baby again, and I hoped that we would succeed. I had been diligently monitoring my LH surge, and then one day it was a "5," so I was "surging." Jeff and I had had such a nice day that if I did conceive, I told myself, I wanted to remember everything about it. It was a Saturday, and Jeff worked up in my study, while I sat in the living room at the cherry desk, reading student papers. Then, when he hadn't appeared by noon, I went out into the beautiful day for a walk. It was the end of February and in the high thirties, not windy for a change, and I walked around Lake Harriet near our house. I had applied in the fall to Ragdale, a writers' and artists' retreat near Chicago, and I was getting excited about going for two weeks in March. I thought about Ragdale and about how I had just gotten a form rejection for a story I had sent out. Rejection seemed inevitable in a writing career. Still, I was glad I had written the story, and I would send it out again. I enjoyed walking along, thinking of these things.

There were many people out, partaking of what

was for Minnesotans an almost-spring day, some even having a picnic and cooking out near the bandstand, as if it were summer! Some college-age boys in bathing suits with their shirts off sat in lawn chairs on what was left of the lake ice near shore. Farther out on the lake, the ice was breaking up; they'd removed the warming house. I could almost see the sailboats again. In the summer the blue lake would be dotted with them.

As I was rounding the west shore bend, I saw Jeff coming to meet me, as I had hoped. We walked over to Linden Hills and had lunch at a hole-in-the-wall Chinese restaurant. Then we walked back around the lake, six miles on the day you might be conceived. We came home and made love. We took our time, and I was trying hard to bring you into the world, though I think for Jeff it was just fun. It wasn't as easy for him to think of you as it was for me. I thought he did think of you, certainly, but I didn't think he lived with the thought of you as I did.

I had spoken to my mother the day before, giving her an update on where we were in infertility treatment. It was a relief to be able to talk to her about it. She wanted you, too. We would all love to have you come—there, an invitation. Please come. Come now. I hope you do. *Come!*

What a world I was inviting you into! Just that week I had learned of the death of a good man who had choked on a sandwich at the age of forty-seven. And a seventeen-year-old girl in our neighborhood had committed suicide, her fourth try, her parents practically camping on her door to keep her from it. But they couldn't stop her; she hung herself. I lay in bed while Jeff napped and thought of all the things that could happen to people. Things that could happen to me, or Jeff. To you. To any of us, at any time. It all seemed so scary, so risky—to bring you into something so uncertain as this life. But worth the risk. I thought of what a lovely day we had had: work, the walk, love. I hoped you would like it, this life. I hoped you wanted to enter it. Please come.

We both slept deeply then, waking about five, and went out and did some errands, just the casual things of a late Saturday afternoon. The bagels we bought were so warm and fragrant we sat and ate one at a window table at the bagel shop. Behind us a mother and daughter were engaged in a serious, troubling talk. The daughter, about fourteen, looked defensive, angry, pained, and the mother, firm, serious, concerned. My eyes filled with tears.

We went on to the Italian deli and bought home-made pasta for supper. I wondered if you would like Italian food. I hoped that I was not just making you up. It would be painful for you not to come, but so likely. What would come, most likely, was my period, the shedding of the bed that could have held you.

Gradually the day approached when I was supposed to leave for Ragdale. I had started my period, and now I would ovulate while I was away. I looked forward to not trying this next time. No Clomid this cycle, no Clomid checks every few days, no LH surge testing, no timed intercourse. No waiting. No disappointment.

A few days before I was supposed to leave, I began to get cold feet. Did I really want to drive seven hours and spend two weeks by myself, with nothing to do but write? What, exactly, had I been thinking of? And yet I wanted to do it. Some part of me kept on with this idea, relentlessly. The day before I was to leave, I stood at the kitchen sink, drying a glass, and thought to myself, God! I won't have to stand here at this sink for two whole weeks, and at the same time I was thinking, God! I won't get to stand here for two whole weeks!

It was hard for me to leave Jeff. In fact, I could hardly bear it. I felt again two opposite, passionate feelings: I couldn't bear to leave him, and I had to get away from him. But I knew how he'd hate to come home to an empty house every night and not have anyone—well, *me*—to talk to. I might desire solitude, but that meant he had to have it too. And he let me know, in various ways, that this was not his first choice.

A few minutes before I was actually to leave, I began to come undone. I burst out crying, unable to stand the thought of the empty house Jeff would come home to that night. I felt so responsible for him, for his happiness, which was part of why I had

to go away. Still, I felt I was deserting him. I had
done everything I could to nurture him while I was
away. I had bought a lot of food, things he liked, easy
to fix. I had cooked a chicken the day before so he'd
have a home-cooked dinner the first night I was
away. I had put up spaghetti sauce and turkey din-
ners in microwave containers. I even set a timer on
the lamp in the entryway so he wouldn't have to
come home to a dark house. But no matter what I
did, I couldn't be in two places at once. I couldn't be
at Ragdale, alone, and at home, together. The idea of
missing any nights of our life together pained me.
And yet I chose it.

Jeff put his arms around me as I was crying
there, trying to leave, and said maybe he had made
it too hard on me to go away. But it wasn't really
him; it was me. Not to sleep in the same bed every
night, not to hear his voice except over long distance, and most of all, not to be able to look into his
eyes. There was always this implicit understanding
between us, this thing that was always being said.

Tears were streaming down my face. I felt like a
fool. We both got in our cars, I in the good car, the
Subaru station wagon, and he in the old car, our '78
Honda. He seemed as reluctant to part with the
Subaru as with me. We drove in tandem down the
freeway, and I kept him in sight, until finally we
approached the point at which he'd continue into
town, to work, and I'd head east toward Milwaukee.
I began to weep again. I thought seriously about

following him on into town, giving up the whole idea. I didn't have to do it. I had a choice. I played it out in my mind. It had great appeal. Back home. Unpacking the car. A cup of tea in my own kitchen to settle my fractured nerves. I could call Ragdale, apologize, explain. It could be done. I was trying to see across the traffic into Jeff's eyes. And then we waved, parted, and I sobbed my way onto I-94 east.

But in a very little while, by the time I reached St. Paul actually, I felt fine. In fact, I was already thinking of something else. I had got past the place where we had to part, the place where we practiced some ultimate parting. Now I was on the open road, heading east, alone, alone-oh, and I felt fine. Two whole weeks to myself. I had my own thoughts, and I didn't have to listen to anyone else, even Jeff. I began to remember other road trips I had taken, when I was young and single. I thought of my dear departed Volkswagen camper, and how I had had to climb up to get into it. It had a huge windshield, like a truck or Greyhound bus. I had liked that.

At Ragdale no one would knock on anyone else's door. We were on our own for breakfast and lunch in the communal kitchen downstairs, and then for dinner we'd go over for a big meal cooked by Maria, the Australian cook extraordinaire.

I sat down every morning to write, and naturally the imp of the perverse was with me. I had hoped that at Ragdale the floodgates would open, and I would suddenly be the fluent, verbally gifted, witty, profound writer I always wanted to be. But I was the same halting writer I was at home. It was not easy, and I wondered why anyone would want to be left alone for two weeks with nothing to do but write. I was always making beds that I had to lie in.

But as I settled in, things got better. And I began to get what I wanted and needed. Silence. Solitude. No other voices. I sometimes felt that I could only write when I was alone. It wasn't true, of course, but when I was alone, when I wasn't likely to be interrupted, I knew that special voice I was always waiting to hear, my writing voice, my own true voice, as I thought of it, was more likely to speak. And it had so much to say! So much of the time it was silent. Beyond silent. Gone. I had to court it, honor it, make room for it. I so longed to hear it. The thought that it would never come again terrified me. Most of the time I filled up all the space it needed with other things. Life was mostly other things. But here at Ragdale, it got to speak.

I was writing a short story called "The Bed." It was about a Northern man, a man from a cold climate, a furniture maker, who marries a Southern woman he meets at a furniture convention in High Point, North Carolina. I based the woman on an old friend of mine, a woman I had met when we were living in Tacoma, a Southerner whom I loved for her beautiful honey blond hair and her effervescent ways. I named her Synthia with an "S," for no better reason than that was the name of one of my great-grandmothers. I put in my great-grandfather's bed, from the Civil War era and made with wooden pegs, the bed my parents slept in in Greenville and which I hoped to inherit one day. In the story Synthia has the bed shipped to Minnesota when she marries the furniture maker. Only, he wants them to sleep in what he considers their own bed, a bed he has made from black cherry he has cut and cured himself. You begin to see the problem. I set one scene at the ocean, because I missed it so. I made up a dog named Buster, a mutt who pranced on his long gray legs as if to say I am so happy and proud to be me! One thing I loved about writing was how you got to put in your favorite things. Writing the story reminded me of my father's old cigar box I had as a child, where I kept such stuff as a blue jay feather, embroidery thread, a shiny piece of mica, buttons that were pretty. I thought about putting the cigar box into the story, but I had to stop somewhere.

I began to notice that I was not, by far, the most solitary person there. There was a young woman artist, for example, who would eat her dinner hurriedly, without saying a word, and then disappear. Sometimes I'd see her hurrying across the big lawn, her long black coat flaring out behind her as she returned to her studio. Once I was startled to come upon her sitting alone in the living room, sipping a cup of something hot in the dark. Solitude rose from her like a mist.

By the beginning of the second week I was deep

into my work. I would wake up early, bring a breakfast tray up to my room so I didn't have to speak to
anyone, and move dreamily to my writing. There
was nothing to distract me, nothing to interrupt me,
nothing to stop me. I spent whole days in blessed
solitude. In blessed work.

14

Dr. Kuneck had introduced the idea of artificial insemination at our last conference. It would ensure that the sperm got past the cervix, since it would be inserted directly into the uterus. Amazingly, I learned, Jeff's sperm would be "cleaned" of debris (debris?) and supercharged with my estrogen. It might give us a better chance, Dr. Kuneck said. But I didn't want to get my hopes up too much. There was no guarantee that artificial insemination—AI— would bring us any nearer to a child.

Jeff and I tried to decide when I got back from Ragdale whether to continue with AI, or quit. "We aren't really equipped to make these godlike decisions," Jeff said. "The best we can do is blunder through."

Work was going better for Jeff. In fact, he had suddenly gotten very busy. He had a big brief due in one case and was taking a deposition in another. A client had come in to give an affidavit, and Jeff had hoped that he'd pay his past due. We needed money, and it wasn't coming in very fast. We were borrowing from our line of credit at the bank; insurance, which we were now paying for ourselves, was covering my infertility treatment.

We decided we would go ahead and try artificial insemination. It made me a little sad to move on to this "unnatural" way. I had had some ridiculous romantic idea about a child being conceived in passion. The chances of my getting pregnant still seemed to me slight; I had run out of time, basically. Still, I didn't want to lose hope right when we were trying something new. It was a hard balancing act, trying to be realistic about my chances and also maintain enough hope even to try.

When my LH surge occurred, I called the clinic for the AI appointment. Jeff was to go in two and a half hours before me because his sperm had to be washed and put in a medium from my blood to activate it more, before being injected into me. I had already had blood drawn, so Jeff went in at a quarter past eight on Friday morning and masturbated in an exam room with a much fingered copy of an old *Playboy* the clinic kept in a briefcase with other dirty magazines, while people milled around talking in the outer office beyond the examination room door. Then I went in two and a half hours later to get inseminated. Jeff went with me; I wanted him there. The procedure was unpleasant to some extent, because Sandy, the nurse who did the insemination, had to clamp my cervix to straighten it out and get the catheter past the inner os. It didn't feel great, and I felt a little full, crampy, after the insemination.

Jeff was quite interested in the whole procedure, and he and Sandy had a jokey time of it, while I lay there with my hips cranked up, feeling a little lonely.

For the next two weeks I tried not to let my imagination run away with me, not to get my hopes up. I knew—I really *knew*—that it probably wouldn't work. But it was hard. Every time we introduced a new element into treatment, my hopes shot way up, only gradually to descend as time passed, and I didn't get pregnant. My nipples did feel sensitive, one of the early signs of pregnancy, but really, they were almost always like that after I ovulated, and Dr. Kuneck had said I wouldn't be able to tell. The truth was there was nothing to do but wait.

One night Jeff asked me when I was supposed to start my period; it was on his mind, too. Normally he didn't think much about when I'd start. But now he was sucked in, in spite of himself. I tried to rein myself in, but it was hard. There was just the waiting, and wondering. One night I had a dream, of a handful of confetti thrown up in the air. Did the dream mean I was pregnant? Did my subconscious *know*? I felt I was working very hard at getting pregnant, inside, and yet there was really very little I could do.

A few nights later I had several bad dreams. I had had a rough night of stomach trouble, which was distressing. I dreamed that my father died, and I was so sad, so disturbed. Then later I had a very angry dream about my mother. I dreamed she grabbed me by the back of my neck, and I thought to myself in the dream, with a lot of hatred, *It's going to take me a long time—if ever—to forgive you for this!* Then the dream skipped to a part about packing to go away, to run away. That had been my way of dealing with my rage at my mother's power and control: to get away.

When I told Lauren about the dreams, she said the one about my mother brought to her mind the image of a mother cat holding a kitten by its neck. I could see the maternal image, but I said it felt to me much fiercer, like an eagle with a mouse and that what the image said to me was, *I'll break your neck if you make a move.* And of course I had made a move. I had made a move, in fact, all the way across the country. It occurred to me that the line from the dream, the line *It's going to take me a long time to forgive you for this!* could have been spoken just as easily by my mother as by me.

My temperature dropped a few tenths of a degree, which meant I'd be starting my period. But then the next day it was back up. I felt I was being toyed with. It was my forty-first birthday. Mama and Daddy called to wish me happy birthday.

I didn't want to get in the same bad way of thinking I might be pregnant as I had before Christmas, but I couldn't seem to help myself. I couldn't believe I was doing it again. But I couldn't control myself. Something bigger than me was in charge, and I resented it.

Finally my period started, and I was much better. At least the uncertainty was over. It was those last couple of days that were the hardest. I always built up a crescendo of nerves and depression and hope and expectation prior to my period. Actually starting was something of a relief. At least I *knew*.

I was correcting the galleys for my book, and blurbs for it were coming in. It was May, and I was working in my garden, getting ready to redo a bed. We began yet another round of Clomid, and when the LH surge test showed I was positive, we scheduled a second round of artificial insemination for the Sunday of Memorial Day weekend. We had rented a rototiller so Jeff could break up the ground for the new flower bed I wanted to put in. He went in on Sunday morning at seven forty-five to make his contribution, and when he came back he began tilling a section of the backyard for me. I was worried about the clematis that grew on the back fence. It was near where Jeff was plowing through the hard dirt, so I told him to be careful not to disturb it. I was standing there warning him about it, and he ran right over it. It was an accident of course, but still! I was furious and I told him so, but there wasn't even time to fight because I had to go in for artificial insemination. He offered to go with me but the novelty had worn off, and I told him he didn't need to.

It was the thirty-first day of my cycle, and I hadn't started my period yet. But I'd been fooled before, several times, and I was no longer as much of a sucker. I reminded myself that just because my temperature hadn't dropped didn't mean I was pregnant. If anything, I felt I would start my period at any moment. But I no longer trusted my feelings about my body. I understood that I couldn't tell.

I was starting a summer school course the next day, so I went to the University to run off some material for the first class, and then I went to Bachman's Garden Center. For an hour or so I wandered around in complete absorption. Everything else fell away as I went row by row looking over the impatiens and geraniums, the delphiniums, dianthus, foxglove, yarrow, hostas, ferns, and lilies.

I began my summer school class on a 93-degree day, in the hottest classroom imaginable. I still hadn't started my period, but I put it out of my mind. I had twenty-three new students to meet, and the first class was always hard for me. It was difficult to believe I'd ever get to know, let alone like, these people. Who were they, and what did they have to do with me? Twenty-three strangers, young people mostly, who wanted to write.

I still hadn't started on the thirty-third day, and now I was beginning to think I might actually be pregnant. I tried not to think about it. I tried to wait, even a few more hours, before going in for a pregnancy test. I felt excited but cautious. I called the clinic to let them know I appeared to be missing my period. They wanted me to come in for a pregnancy test. I told myself I probably wasn't pregnant, but I indulged in looking up when the baby would be born — *if I were pregnant, and if everything went okay*: February 19.

Driving over to get the pregnancy test, I thought about how I used to believe being pregnant meant you'd have a child. Now I thought it meant you'd have a blighted ovum. But my mother had had two successful pregnancies. Lots of women did. Maybe I could, too. It occurred to me that my doubts were more or less resolved. Given the choice between having a child and not having one, I'd have one. But I also thought that I could live without having one. On the front seat I had a bag of muffins, a treat I was taking in for the staff.

Linda called me a little after two that afternoon. The pregnancy test is positive, she exclaimed. You're pregnant! *Pregnant?* I stuttered back to her. *That's amazing!* But I could hardly believe it. I was thrilled — but — could it work? I called Jeff immediately, and told him the news, and he said he was thrilled too, but we were both a little stunned. It seemed like such a monumental thing, and at the same time so little — a few cells beginning to multiply. I had always heard that you couldn't be just a little bit pregnant, but now I realized that you could. I called home, and my mother was at the beauty parlor. I told my father, and heard how his voice filled up with tears. Then I called Jeff's parents, and left a message on the phone answering machine. When I hung up, I hardly knew what to do.

It was late afternoon, and I still had to teach that night. I was pregnant at last, but life went on. In fact, I needed to keep preparing my notes. I wrote down some thoughts for the class, trying to get organized.

Ahhhhh! *Pregnant.*

I had my first doctor's appointment. Everyone at the office was excited. Dr. Kuneck came in and shook my hand and said he was "thrilled," but also, we couldn't dance on the top of the desk yet. I was still in the "chemical phase" and my chances of miscarriage were 30–40 percent.

Several weeks passed, and I was still pregnant. My blood work showed everything progressing well, and everywhere I went, and everything I did, I carried with me the knowledge, the beautiful secret, that I was pregnant.

I began to tell people about the pregnancy. Dr. Kuneck had warned me against telling while it was still so early, but I felt wonderful, happy to be pregnant. I couldn't imagine not telling my friends, many of whom knew about my infertility treatment. I was enjoying being a pregnant person. I had always wanted to eat for two. I didn't have any nausea, any morning sickness. In fact, I felt wonderful.

I began, begrudgingly, to like my students, the usual course. I felt a certain incipient affection for them. And I was fascinated that now when I taught the class, I was pregnant.

Jeff had a dream. He was at the hospital, where he had gone to see our baby. And there it was, laughing and smiling. Everyone was gathered around to see such a happy baby.

Dr. Kuneck scheduled my first ultrasound for the coming week. He wanted to see if the pregnancy was actually in the uterus, and by now, he told me, they might see a heartbeat.

The night before the ultrasound I had a restless sleep. I dreamed that I had forgotten to take the water to drink before the test, and I had to come back to the house. In the bathroom, I saw Creepy, long dead, but in the dream he had never been gone, so I felt a little confused about why I was so happy to see him again. And then Cecil came in, and the three of us were in that little space, and I was so happy to be with the cats again. Then I woke up, disturbed. I couldn't figure out the dream. Could it possibly mean that I might have twins? I decided I'd love to have twins.

Jeff went with me for the ultrasound. I lay on a table with my pants off, and Chad, the ultrasound technician, a person of delicate sensibilities given the circumstances, had me insert a probe into my vagina. We watched as my uterus came onto the screen, like a weather map, and then we saw it, the dark spot, the fetal sac, there, where it should be, and while Chad took measurements and pictures of it, Jeff and I gazed and gazed.

Dr. Kuneck came in. He stared at the screen. He told us that at this stage, in 70 percent of the cases, we'd be able to see the heartbeat. But maybe it was not mature enough yet, and I should come back next week. We'd see. I tried not to think about it. All I could do was wait and see. We still felt lucky. Hopeful.

15

It is hard to receive bad news in public. It is hard, of course, to receive it in private, but in public, one feels (*I* feel) the need to maintain some composure, the semblance of being able to handle it.

I was lying on the examination table in the ultrasound room a week later with the probe inserted into my vagina, only this time the technician was a woman, or a girl, as I thought of her, and not a person of Chad's sensitivities. Jeff was in federal court, trying a case, and it hadn't occurred to me to ask someone else to come with me. I thought of myself as braced for bad news.

I'd been there forty minutes now, and I was bored with the whole thing. My neck had a crick in it from trying to stare at the monitor to my right, and in some way, I didn't even care anymore. I looked at the ceiling. I couldn't get any answers out of this girl. She deferred to the doctor, naturally— "he'll have to be the one to say"—and I shrugged, wondering what I would do in her situation, what I would say. I'd like to think I'd come out with it. The truth. Dr. Kuneck arrived, grave in the darkened room, and I didn't even look at the screen anymore. I was not in suspense. I wanted to go home. He and the technician stared at the screen for a long time. Finally I said, impatient, "Well, what do you see?"

Now it came: words that both surprised me and yet seemed familiar, as if I'd already heard them. "Do you want me to give it to you straight," he said, and with those words, he already had.

There was a flurry—a scurry—on the part of the lab technician. She wanted to get out of there fast. Then we were alone. I sat up. Of course I do, I said in a firm voice. So he said it: I don't believe at this point that the pregnancy is viable.

The world went on, I sat there, we talked a few minutes, some statistics, his favorite thing, were tossed about, and he said he'd see me in his office in a few moments. Then I was alone. I got up and put back on my clothes. I wandered out into the hall, and someone came up to me, and told me to sit in that chair, to wait for the report that I would carry down to my doctor's office. I started toward the chair, but then the person said, No, why don't you go on down, and we'll send it. Had they seen something that I couldn't see? Something about me.

I knew that I had my eyes open, and I found my way down the corridors of the hospital that I knew so well, but I was like a blind person. Something was wrong, and it seemed to be in me, it seemed to be building in me, but at the same time, I couldn't quite feel it, I couldn't see it. It was growing. By the time I reached my doctor's office, I was filled to the brim with it. I pushed open the door, and Linda, who just a few weeks ago said so brightly over the phone, "You're going to have a little Southern Belle, or Beau!" now spoke one word: my name. I stood by the reception desk. I had the idea that I could not go into the waiting area and take a chair, and I felt that if I stood there, which was as far as I had been able to get, Dr. Kuneck would see me right away. Linda was coming around the desk to me, and suddenly I realized I couldn't wait, I had to get out to my car, because the feeling, whatever it was, was over-whelming me. I tried to say to her: *I better make an appointment and come back.* That was clearly what I wanted to say, something simple and easy, it made sense to me, but I was unable to speak. I tried to get these words out, and I couldn't tell if I was succeed-ing. Then, before I knew it, a terrible sob ripped out of me. It had a life of its own, it was out of my con-trol, and the "I" I thought I knew dissolved in the face of this awful sound, I was reduced to this horri-ble, wrenching Sob. The "I" I used to know, the "I" I counted on, thought briefly of the other people around me—there were several, other patients, peo-ple I sensed on the periphery of the Sob—but that "I" could care no more, for the Sob was everything, the Sob was what was real now, with its big need, taking up the whole world.

It is good to break down in public. It gives other people a chance to be kind, and it can show you, finally, that you're not so alone.

Linda led me down the hall. I marveled, from far away, inside the Sob, that she knew just what to do. She sat me down, and I gave in, briefly, to the sobbing. She stood next to me, and put her arm around me, and the side of my face was pressed into the blue polyester of her hip. I was surprised at myself. I was filled with wonder. This was the end of control, and the beginning of something else. Linda told me she understood and then she told me her own story, how she had had a miscarriage herself, and how after that she had a baby who died shortly after birth. This stopped me in my tracks. I turned and looked up at her, her pale poignant face. My own loss seemed small in the light of this. Smaller. I was filled with sympathy for her, which took my mind off my own sympathy for myself, a relief. I could not stay here and bawl, nor did I want to. I loved Linda because she did understand, she understood too well; I wished I could spare her such knowledge. I began to calm down.

When Linda left, Patty came in, darling Patty, with her big red glasses, so kind and gentle, motherly in the best way, with two little adopted children of her own. She was so sorry for me, and to tell the truth, I was sorry for me, too. She got me a cold drink, she wrung out a cold washcloth and held it to my face. When Patty left, Sandy came in, the one who artificially inseminated me, full of kind words, and when she left Dr. Kuneck came in. He was troubled, saddened, taking it hard. I felt I should comfort him.

But now I was in a fix. I was carrying a nonviable pregnancy, and I had to get rid of it, one way or another. We could wait until I aborted naturally, or I could have a D & C. I could have a miscarriage at any time, he told me, and I realized that as often as I'd heard about miscarriages, I had no idea what one was like. I was to call him if I started bleeding or cramping. I thought of having the miscarriage while I was teaching, in front of my now-dear students. What if I had to lie down on the classroom floor? I opted for the D & C, but I fretted about timing. I wanted to finish teaching my class. All the final papers were coming in next week. We scheduled for two days after I finished the class. I went home carrying a paper bag, inside of which was a clear plastic jar with some saline solution in it.

This moment, then: I gaze. I gaze. I gaze at the dark spot on the ultrasound screen. I am lying there covered with a sheet, my pants off, the probe stuck into me, moved this way and that by Chad, and Jeff is there, it is the first ultrasound, the one before the bad news, the one where it is still too soon to be sure there is no heartbeat, that will come next week, but this week, I gaze. I gaze at the dark spot on the screen, my developing pregnancy. It is there, absolutely unmistakable, though mysterious too, unreadable, a spot on the moon, a dark crater we see but cannot know. My pregnancy. Not a baby, certainly not that—it will never get that far. It will never be a baby I lose; it will be a pregnancy. Still, something precious to me, something resisted, longed for, fought for, celebrated—this dark spot on the ultrasound screen, this moment when I turn my head and gaze. When it is finally—there. There it is. I gaze at it. I hold it in my eyes.

I am trying to wake up from the D & C. Someone is speaking to me: Dr. Kuneck. *"Everything went well. You are all right."* I try to speak to him, to thank him, but I am so deep I cannot bring my voice to the surface. Instead, I grope for his hand and squeeze it.

Now I become the sad receptacle of miscarriage stories. Women bring them to me, in sympathy and comfort, like flowers.

It is a few weeks after the D & C. Dr. Kuneck has scheduled an appointment for us with the geneticist who has studied what he removed. I want to know what has gone wrong, and if it is age related. She holds up pictures of chromosomes, the familiar twenty-three pairs, and points out the twentieth pair, the pair that in our case had the nondisjunction, the pair that did us in. She tells us the egg would have been defective all along, that the good eggs tend to go first.

She talks on and on, but I come to when she refers to "her." Her? I think. Who?

That's right, she says. It—of course there was no fetus yet—the tissue—had two X chromosomes. It would have been a girl.

III

16

"After great pain," Emily Dickinson wrote, "a formal feeling comes—." Those words came back to me that summer after I lost the pregnancy. I didn't feel I had lost a child, though some women do feel that after a miscarriage. But I did feel the loss of a lot of possibility. I had been headed in one direction with great momentum, only to be pulled up short, and I felt, if not lost, at least disoriented, uncertain which way to go. Although I "understood" what had happened, the loss of that pregnancy—and all it took with it—felt too big to encompass, so I had to settle for a formal feeling.

The summer passed, then, in a kind of meditation, a reckoning of sorts. I put in the new garden, took walks around the lake, postponed any decisions about trying again. I was in an interstice—there was nothing I had to do, nothing I had to decide. I sat at my desk and wrote. I didn't see how anyone got through life without writing. When we made love for the first time after the D & C, I wept. And even though I didn't want to, I couldn't help thinking,

Maybe I'll get pregnant again. Maybe even tonight . . .
But I also knew I wasn't ready to take it on again.

In August my parents and Aunt Grace and Uncle Perry came to Minnesota, and we took them to Jeff's parents' cabin in northern Wisconsin. The visit was full of fragile, poignant moments, such as trying to get those four old ones into Jeff's father's boat. They all wanted to go for a ride, but what had been simple and easy when they were young was now a major production. Everything moved in slow motion, and I had to turn away as Jeff helped them, for fear one of them would fall between the dock and the boat. But off we finally went, my father and Uncle Perry up front, tiny old men in feed caps, and my mother and aunt huddled in the back with net bonnets on to keep their hairdos from blowing. After we put them all on the plane back to South Carolina, I turned to Jeff in relief and said, "It must have been a success. No one died."

Then in September, *Feeding the Eagles* was released. It was out, in public, in the world. Sheila Murphy, the marketing director at Graywolf, called me from their offices in St. Paul: "Two of them just walked in the door." It was a Friday afternoon, and Jeff and I were planning to go to the North Shore for the weekend. It took us a while to get ready, and all the time we were packing, I felt astonished: in a little while I'd be seeing my book for the first time.

We drove over to St. Paul, with me in a nervous, excited state. When we walked into the Graywolf offices, Sheila came out and handed me the book. Scott and the rest of the staff gathered around. I took it in my hands. It was a dark rich green, with an original chalk drawing of a cabin at dusk reproduced on the front. I turned it over and read the dust jacket blurbs. One was from Wallace Stegner, who had been so kind to me at Stanford, and who was being kind still. I thanked the Graywolf staff, but mainly I wanted to get away, to be alone with it. I couldn't absorb it in public.

Then Jeff and I were driving north, and I sat there turning it over and over in my hands.

That night in our cabin beside Lake Superior, I sat up late. I examined the book's every detail. I tried to see how it might seem to a reader, someone I didn't know, someone who bought it and who didn't know me. I thought it was all right. I couldn't tell if it was actually good. But mainly I couldn't get over the book's physical reality: the ISBN, the solid heft of it in my hands.

I thought about how each story came out of some core of pain, some sense of loss that only writing could assuage. I had wanted to capture the people and places I loved and move them outside of time. The main character in my collection—Miriam—was described as the kind of person who does not like to let go. I was trying to hold on to what time and life itself were removing from me. I felt, underneath the surface of everything, the gaping chasm of loss and death. Writing was my way of fighting back. My parents were growing old; I was aware that they would not always be with me. I wanted them to live in my book, forever. I wrote about a beloved cabin we had to sell, and I knew that in describing that place—the couches covered in brown and white material, the fieldstone fireplace, the three wire ducks over the mantel, the curtains of red my mother made—that I would have our cabin forever, if not in reality then in language. It would always be there, in my book, for me to return to.

When I was eighteen I had four impacted wisdom teeth removed. I had never had any kind of operation before, and this procedure required my being put to sleep. I was afraid I wouldn't wake up. But of course the procedure went fine and I did wake up. As I was coming to, rising to the surface from what felt like a very dark hole of unconsciousness, I had a revelation: I believed in literature. I meant this in the same way that people believe in God. It was a private thing, something I never mentioned to anyone. I couldn't explain it anymore than someone can explain their love of God, their need for Him. But there it was. I believed in literature, it became my religion and for all these years, in my own frail way, I had been true to it.

I sat with the book on my lap, my hands resting on it lightly. How far I had traveled to arrive at this moment! How tenaciously I had clung to this goal. Was it worth it? For me it was, absolutely. It gave me deep pleasure to have written those stories, to be a small tributary feeding the great ocean of literature, to have beat back death. It felt wonderful to have accomplished what I had wanted to do for so long.

But I also knew it had cost me. I was forty-one years old and I didn't have a child. In college I had written a paper for sociology called "Women as Writers" in which I pondered all the reasons why so much more literature seemed (back then) to be written by men than women. I was under the influence of Virginia Woolf's *A Room of One's Own*, and a lesser-known work by Margaret Lawrence called *The School of Femininity*. Even as a junior in college I had been convinced that a great danger to a woman who wanted to be a writer was getting married and having babies. I had said something in the paper along the lines of "One can only conjecture about how many great feminine novels are walking around in flesh and blood. Women seem to have babies instead of books." From the very start, I had seen writing and motherhood as mutually exclusive.

Now when I looked around me, most of the women writers I knew had children. They even wrote articles and books about it, counteracting the very notion that had seemed a hard truth in the late sixties, when I was writing my college paper. Women, we had come to understand, did not have to choose. They could do both—at least a lot of them could. Maybe I could have. But I remembered how it had been back then, the dark ages, at the very dawn of the women's movement in the sixties. It had been a man's world in a way that was hard to believe today.

I thought again of that long ago time when I had

said no not only to Bill Nelson's parents' French Provincial living room furniture but to everything else that I felt was expected of me—all the female roles that had seemed at the time so diametrically opposed to becoming a writer. I wondered about the beliefs and boundaries we devise for our own lives. I felt now that if I had had children earlier, I would simply have found out about myself in different ways. I might not have had writing; for me that still felt like a truth. But I couldn't be sure. There were so many ways to be a woman, wife, mother, writer. I had had to relinquish some things in order to get others. But I had wanted this book. I might also want other things—I certainly did—but I had gotten one thing that I had to have.

Graywolf was hosting a publication party for me the next week. The day of the party, flowers began arriving at the house, and Jeff gave me a beautiful glass eagle. In the title story of the book, Miriam and Ted, her husband, are out in a boat on a Wisconsin lake. Ted catches a big Northern, which he throws back, but it floats to the surface, and an eagle suddenly swoops down and carries it away. It was an image having to do with the cycles of life, how death and life are intertwined. "You don't have to feel so bad," Ted says to Miriam about the fish's death. "We're feeding the eagles." I sat the glass eagle on the buffet in the dining room, where its strength and dignity could watch over us.

I couldn't eat dinner before the party. I was extraordinarily nervous, almost to the point where I couldn't speak. I wondered how I would manage to read the story I planned to read, which was about my father losing his radio and TV store on North Main Street. But once I arrived I felt very calm and self-possessed. I opened the book and began to read. Then, miraculously, I was seated at a table, signing books.

I couldn't get to sleep that night until after three, and then I woke at five. So many people I knew and loved had come to the publication party. I had to go over every detail in my mind.

I drove over to Odegard's bookstore the next day, to see if the book was in stock. Its gorgeous green self was in the window—a whole display of them. I could see how easy it would be for a book to get lost among all the others in a store. I wanted mine to hold its own, to find its way in the world.

I wanted to write another book. Then another. I wanted to sit at my desk and write. And I thought, not for the first time, but with more confidence, that the only way to succeed at writing is to be absolutely true to what is your own.

17

Several months had passed since the pregnancy, and I didn't know whether we should try again. I could tell by my calendar that I was approaching my fertile time. But I didn't feel very fertile. Since I wasn't taking Clomid anymore, I had probably reverted back to the luteal phase problem, which meant even if I did get pregnant, I wouldn't be able to sustain it. No one could answer the question for me of whether or not it was time to give up.

I decided to go to a Resolve meeting again. I wanted to see how our case would sound, out loud, in public. I wanted to know whether there were any cracks in the argument I was making to myself, that it was too late.

The meeting was held in the fellowship room of a Lutheran church. I had been there once before, a long time ago. I was just getting started then with infertility treatment, and I had not faced that I might not be able to give birth to a child. I had taken the name "Resolve" to mean "will," as in, you resolve to have a child, you put your will to it, and you succeed. But now I understood it differently: resolve, as in resolution. Closure.

There were several people there. The couple who sat across from me was young and sexy. She was good looking in a loose way, like a teenager, though she was perhaps thirty. She chewed gum the whole time and had a "give me a break" way of talking. She wore black pedal pushers that exposed her smooth tan calves and little black pumps with colored rhinestones. Her husband was so good-looking I tried not to stare. He wore baggy pants, smoky blue, that made me think of his sex. They sat on a couch together, snuggled very close, like two beautiful children. They never, during the whole meeting, released one another.

The other couple was as unattractive and unsexual as the first was attractive and sexual. It depressed me to look at them. The woman had plain brown hair cut short and a clean scrubbed face with pale bulging eyes behind nondescript glasses. Her clothes were functional, they covered her body. He wore blue jeans and a white shirt, and I forgot his face the moment I looked away from him.

Of the other women there, one was terribly pretty, fragile, sympathetic; another, lively, deep-voiced, and ungrammatical; and the third I took an immediate dislike to. She was loud and bossy, with all her facial features crowded toward the middle. Infertility was her career. She had seen it all, done it all, had it all, and knew it all. She had signed up for life in the Infertility Wars.

The leader of the group had resolved her own

infertility by adopting a little girl from China. It wasn't as if I wasn't aware of adoption. But I wanted to be pregnant, to have our own child, a child that came from Jeff and me. Adoption, at least at the moment, did not seem to be a solution to the problem that I had.

When it came my turn to talk, I told them I was trying to come to terms with not being able to have a child. And I was having a hard time with it. I didn't want to cry, though I knew the people in that room were well acquainted with tears.

When I got home I told Jeff about the meeting. I had gone hoping that something would become clearer. I told how no one had tried to talk me out of stopping—though I wished they had. I had gone, I now realized, hoping someone would say, "It's not too late! Don't stop now!" But no one had said that, and how, after all, could they? I still felt, I told Jeff, that I had come to the end of trying to have a child. I was too old. It was too late. It might be hard, but it had to be done. Then I went and stood in a hot shower, and tried to let the hot water leach out some of the pain.

A few nights later I dreamed that I had lost my cat Charlotte. In the dream Charlotte was pure white. In real life she had been a handsome black Persian with white markings. I never saw her in the dream—she was already gone. I tore through the dream house, searching for Charlotte. The irrefutable truth was impressing itself on me, like news of a death. Charlotte was gone, and nothing would bring her back.

An enormous grief was welling in me, an inconsolable despair. Something — someone — infinitely precious to me, loved beyond reason — could not be recovered. It took the form of a white cat. I was so inconsolable that I woke up.

And knew at once that the dream was about losing a child, or more precisely, losing the hope of having a child. This truth spoke to me with complete certainty.

I was on day twenty-six of my cycle. I expected to start my period in a day or two. Perhaps the dream resulted from some shift in my hormones. Perhaps as the estrogen and progesterone levels fell, in preparation for menstruation, my brain grew alarmed and formed the dream of the missing cat, a dream that told me I was not ready to give up.

Deciding to try again, I felt happy. I had undergone a miraculous cure. All the pain I had been feeling disappeared. I did not have to give up on having a child. Hope came back, tender and green. Jeff wanted to try again, too, he said. Everything seemed simple. It might not be too late. I had gotten pregnant once. I could get pregnant again. It still might work out.

We decided on a game plan. We would try for six more months, six more months of Clomid and artificial insemination. It was nothing, really, compared to what a lot of people go through, but it was still hard for me. Infertility treatment is not something to prolong lightly. Six tries were supposed to be enough, statistically. After six months, if I wasn't pregnant, we'd reassess. That was the word we used: *reassess*. We weren't closing any doors, and we wouldn't have to decide, month in and month out, what to do.

Graywolf was sending me clippings of reviews, and one was (oddly, I thought) from *Business Week*: "By focusing on the transformational powers of loss, and the restorative power of memory, Alden conveys the sense that loss and gain are merely opposite faces of the same, indivisible coin." I studied this quote. That gains and losses were opposite faces of the same, indivisible coin was a lesson I had to learn over and over, and the way I tried to teach it to myself was through writing.

The first month went by. The second. The third. Fourth. Fifth. Sixth. They went by that fast, like snaps of the fingers.

Reassessment. We sat in Dr. Kuneck's office and heard the possibilities: keep on with what we were doing, Clomid and artificial insemination; escalate the treatment by taking Pergonal injections to hyperstimulate my ovaries (*hyperstimulate my ovaries?*); move to a high-tech procedure like GIFT (gamete intrafallopian transfer); or come to closure.

"Am I your oldest patient?"

Dr. Kuneck looked at me with some surprise.

"Why, no," he said. "I have two patients who are forty-two who are pregnant."

I didn't know whether to consider this good news or bad.

"Well, then, how old is your oldest patient?"

"Forty-eight."

I put my head down on his desk and beat it softly.

Now, I decided, we were really through. It was *really* time to stop. We had tried six more times, and nothing had happened. Six more months of rising hope and crashing disappointment. Didn't that tell us something? I had turned forty-two, and surely now I was too old. I needed to get to the end of all this, but I didn't know how.

Jeff and I began to tell each other that actually, it was pretty nice not trying anymore, and that really, we liked our life the way it was. I can see us at sixty, Jeff speculated one day, not with a kid beginning college, but traveling, writing, having a good life. Immediately, strangely, an image of us on a cruise ship came to my mind. Jeff and me on a cruise ship? And then I wondered, would I be sixty and leaning over the rail of a cruise ship feeling sad that I had never had a child?

It was true that I had moments of actual mourning. This is what grief is like, I thought, how it breaks you and breaks you and then breaks you again. I walked around the lake one day with Sasha, and when she asked me what I was writing, I said a piece

called "On Not Having a Child." That's pretty defini-
tive, she said, and I remember how at that point in
our walk I looked around me and the whole scene —
the lake, the trees, the path, the sky — was suffused
with loss.

I figured that time would help. I concentrated
on putting days under my belt. I wanted to have
the issue of a child behind me, to have it settled,
done. To be normal again. I wanted my old self back,
though I suspected, with fear, that I was never to be
my old self again. I knew it was not tragic not to
have a child. But I couldn't seem to get over feeling
tragic. I'd spend the summer healing, I told myself,
and then in the fall, I would be all right.

I made a point of talking to women who did not
have children, but had wanted them. They told me
that there was life after the pain of not having a
child. Life, they told me, definitely goes on. Your cells
adjust, one poet friend told me. "Let's talk clichés,"
she said brightly. "There are apples and there are
oranges, and I want to be the best orange I can be."
I thought I knew, somewhat, what she meant. She
was happy and content with her life now. She had
finally realized, she said, that not having children
was actually what was right for her. I gazed at her
with admiration and envy, but she was speaking
from a place I could only as yet imagine.

Maybe I will arrive at that feeling someday, I
thought. Maybe I will be at peace. I pictured a more
mature, wiser self, someone who had been to battle,

fought a good fight, and was now retired. Someone who had let go of one thing in order to have
other things. Someone who had grieved, and then
moved on.

But for now it was the Summer of Babies. Everywhere I went I picked up stories of infertility, births,
miscarriages, pregnancies, adoptions. The whole world
seemed involved in a gigantic spasm of procreation,
and I couldn't escape.

My sister-in-law, Mary Ellen, was seven months
pregnant. I had thought I couldn't live through her
first pregnancy, and now she was pregnant again. I
had particular trouble with babies in the family,
calling up as they did all my own feelings of lack of
family. But Peter and Mary Ellen were preparing to
leave for his year's residency in vascular surgery in
St. Louis. We hadn't seen them in several months,
and I wanted to have them over to say good-bye, to
wish them well on their next adventure. I dreaded
seeing Mary Ellen—the sight of that swollen, fertile
belly—but that didn't overcome my affection for
her. And I both wanted and didn't want to see our
little nephew John.

It didn't work out too badly. I hugged Mary Ellen,
took in her big belly, and lived. And as for the baby,
he was not excruciatingly cute, as I must have fantasized, living as I did in an almost totally childless
world. He was simply a very active, curious, pleasant
little boy who kept us all hopping during dinner. He
dominated for the simple fact that he was eighteen

months old, and not in his own home. Someone had to be after him all the time, otherwise he was opening the cabinet under the sink, dumping the can of Drano upside down, pulling open the china cabinet doors, or climbing the stairs. We took turns during dinner getting up from the table to occupy him, and I noticed that it did not occur to Jeff that he might take a turn. Maybe it *was* just as well that we hadn't had a child. On my watch, I followed John up the stairs, which he mounted with amazing speed, and stood by, tall and awkward, while he pushed the rocking chair in our bedroom back and forth a few hundred times, and pointed to the ceiling fan and said "fa, fa," which I repeated back to him in an idiotic way.

When they left, at nine, exhausted, I had to admit that perhaps my moaning and groaning about not having a child was taking place in some realm removed from reality. I tried to imagine my quiet life of writing and reading with an eighteen-month-old. I saw that some major adjustments would have to be made. I could make them, no doubt, as other women did, but it would cost me. It would cost me a lot. I had always known, deeply, that having a child came with a price, especially for women, and I had just caught a glimpse of the tag.

Meanwhile my friend Jennifer was still pregnant. In fact, she was very pregnant. I was shocked, because I was so used to Jennifer having miscarriages.

In the past two years or so she had had four. It was taking me a while to get it into my head that this pregnancy was actually going to work. But now, clearly, things were going full steam ahead. She was decorating a baby room, going hog-wild on Bellini furniture.

I wanted to buy a baby gift and take Jennifer out for a special luncheon to celebrate the baby. I felt guilty that I couldn't give her a shower, but I just couldn't. I had turned down several invitations to baby showers that summer, but I didn't want to let the approach of Jennifer's baby go by without some celebration.

I wanted the present to be very special, and I found what I thought was the perfect thing, a baby blanket, a soft cotton weave of blue and white. I was so pleased with it, and pleased with myself for handling the purchase without too much trouble. Baby stores, after all, were not my favorite thing. But when I walked out the door, holding the wrapped gift in a sack, I started to pant. The pain was so sudden and intense it took my breath away.

I told Jennifer I wanted to come over, see the baby's room, take her out to lunch. I had to do it. I wanted to do it. And I knew I could do it, for the simple fact that Jennifer knew all about my own troubles, and she would not deny them. I wouldn't have asked you to see the baby's room, she said, but since you asked. We stood in the lovely room, with its perfect new furniture, crib and changing table, a rocker in the light from the window, the anticipation of a new life.

I loved Jennifer because she never for a minute forgot, she never for a minute pretended that things weren't the way they were for me. We talked about it. We both had tears. We also had a very good lunch, Chinese chicken salad. We were good women friends, and like good women friends we took turns: what was going on in my life, what was going on in hers.

Jennifer and Mary Ellen both had their babies the last week of August, and I started my period. I had a long talk with Jeff. "Where have you been in all this?" I was plagued by the idea that he hadn't really been present in some way during all our efforts to have a child. He had been wonderful, he had been supportive, he had done all the right things, but in some way I felt alone.

"I think my attitude in life is, Accept what you get, and don't feel pain or disappointment for all you don't get."

I took that in. "What else?" I said.

"You want to have a baby," he said. "I want us to survive infertility."

I nodded my head. I was aware that Jeff was not programmed for reproduction the way I was. That was how I felt at times: as if I were wired, beyond my control. This was curious to me. Maybe biology was destiny, after all. I thought of how I moved in such a female world where periods, pregnancies, babies, bodies were at the core of that world to an extent larger than I had realized. But even if I did feel alone in my obsession, it was a relief to me that Jeff had never been as distraught about it as I had been. How could we have stood two of me?

One night I got a phone call from Jennifer telling me how happy she was, how *content*. "I finally have my family," she said. I was glad for her to tell me what she was feeling; that was, after all, the basis of our friendship. But when I hung up, I was in a dark place. I remembered some lines from Roethke: "Snail, snail, glister me forward, bird, soft sigh me home. Worm, be with me. This is my hard time." I had a few black words with Jeff, unfairly, and then I went to bed, to get rid of myself. During the night it felt as if someone was stomping on my stomach. I was tired of it all. Tired of feeling pain, grief, frustration, confusion, disappointment, loss. All of it. I was seriously tired of it.

The next morning when I went downstairs for breakfast, in the newspaper was a story about a couple who had achieved a child through the GIFT (gamete intrafallopian transfer) program at my infertility clinic at Abbott Northwestern Hospital. In fact, I remembered the very day they had the procedure, in which eggs are retrieved from the ovaries and implanted along with sperm in the fallopian tubes. I had been getting artificial insemination that day (per usual), and Sandy told me they had done a GIFT procedure that morning. And now here they were, their smiling pictures in the newspaper, holding up a baby girl. I read the article through my tears. It was all about how happy they were, how horrible infertility had been, how they had tried for years, never given up, and finally succeeded. Jeff came down, took one look at my face, and said, "Let's try again."

18

I had always wanted to be sensible, reasonable, in control, never to make a mistake, never to get hurt, and my basic stance toward life was cautious, if not downright chicken, so how was it, I wondered, that I found myself, at forty-two years of age, leaning on my elbow on our dresser to take the weight off one foot, my pants pulled partway down, while my husband, a surgeon's son squeamish about anything having to do with blood, steadied himself to stick an inch-and-a-half needle into my hip? How was it, I wondered, that now, at odd moments, Jeff would look at me with a glint in his eye, and say, "Want a shot?" What had seemed to me fantastical, scary, and unacceptable a few months ago—hyperstimulation of my ovaries to produce more eggs, and therefore increase our chances of conceiving—now in the fall seemed entirely desirable. The fact that Jeff was the one to give me the shots—a detail the infertility people considered minor and routine—seemed to us, at least initially, so dramatic and nerve-wracking that we didn't see why it shouldn't work. We were going so much farther, after all, than we had ever dreamed.

We had gone in a few days before the start of my cycle for injection training. Sandy put us in a conference room and turned on a videotape of a woman demonstrating how to mix saline solution with ampules of Pergonal, filling a syringe and giving an intramuscular injection in the upper quadrant of the hip. She spoke so rapidly — "nowyoubreakoffthetopofthe ampuleandthenyouinjecttwocc'sofairintothe . . ." — that we had to keep stopping the videotape and backing it up. I had never heard the word "ampule" before, I had never been on anything but the receiving end of a syringe, and as soon as I uncapped one I stuck myself in the finger. Nervously, unable to believe we'd soon be doing this on our own, we practiced uncapping the needles, attaching them to syringes, drawing up liquid and shooting it slowly into an empty vial of Pergonal, freeze-dried FSH (follicle-stimulating hormone) and LH (luteinizing hormone) extracted, we learned, from the urine of postmenopausal nuns. Then we practiced injecting an orange, which, I realized, would soon be replaced by my backside. Jeff's hands seemed huge, clumsy, and inept. After about an hour of this Sandy came in to see how we were doing, and if we had any questions. Jeff just looked at her funny, and said, "What do we do?"

Finally the evening arrived for the first shot. We were both quite nervous, though I tried to take it philosophically. For some reason it was important for us to be trying again. We had to go this extra mile;

we couldn't finish what wasn't over. Jeff swabbed a spot on my upper hip with a cold alcohol rub; we studied the diagram of where the shot would go. He had to draw air into the vacuum of the vial, and then mix the Pergonal with some saline solution. He looked like a mad scientist, though for once he wasn't joking around. He was supposed to stick it in me a little ways, pull the needle out a bit to check for blood to make sure he wasn't in a vein, and then push it in and slowly inject the solution. Some guys, we had learned, couldn't give the shots. But some women could give them to themselves, in their upper thighs. Finally, counting too quickly to three I thought, he stuck it in, pulled it back quickly, and then gave me the shot. It didn't even hurt that much. It went in so fast, and I was trying so hard not to tense my hip that I was surprised that there was only a quick sting. The only catch was he left the needle in afterward, thinking in a tiz that he had to open a band-aid before he took the needle out. I was shocked to look back and see it still sticking out of me. When he finally pulled it out, and put a band-aid on me, we shook hands. A job well done, or, at least, done.

I was going in several times a times a week now for ultrasounds, so that the staff could monitor how many follicles—the fluid-filled capsules that surround the eggs while they are developing—I was producing, to make sure they weren't getting too big, and to try to predict when they were ready to release an egg, so that we could time insemination then. Jeff was giving me Pergonal shots every night. The first month I only conjured up one follicle, and my estradiol, which was measured through blood work, was only 300. We had started off with the lowest possible dose of Pergonal to see how I would respond—they didn't want to hyperstimulate my ovaries too much, but I had hoped for a few more eggs to give us a better chance. We went ahead with insemination, and then Jeff gave me a series of HCG (human chorionic gonadotropin) shots to help me sustain the pregnancy, should there be one.

All in all I was spending more time than ever at the infertility clinic. There were always other women in the ultrasound waiting room. I knew they were probably on Pergonal, too, and I longed to ask them about their experiences, but I was afraid to break the code of privacy. We never did more than nod at one another, though we recognized each other as patients of Dr. Kuneck. Sometimes as many as eighteen women got ultrasound monitoring on a single day. The ultrasound technicians referred to us as "follicles." "We've got ten follicles to do today."

But Pergonal was not going to be any miracle either. After several rounds, I began to feel again that I was embarked on a futile course. I worried about what such strong drugs were doing to my body, what the long-term effects might be. It bothered me to be keeping on with what I felt was essentially hopeless.

I wondered if I was addicted to infertility treatment. There was such a desire to succeed, not to fail, not to give up. I couldn't believe, in some part of me, that if I wanted a child, my own biological child, I couldn't have one. But I also knew that my chances were slight.

I was in a lonely place. I wasn't teaching that quarter, and I felt odd and isolated. I was spending my mornings getting ultrasounds, and my evenings getting shots, and the rest of the world seemed to be rushing by, procreating effortlessly from what I could tell.

When it was time for another round of insemination, I had three follicles developing. I was so proud of my three little follicles, until Chad told me about the woman he had monitored earlier that morning, who was being prepared for the GIFT program. She had had ten follicles on one side, and fourteen on the other.

It was the weekend, and a new doctor who had joined Dr. Kuneck in his burgeoning infertility practice was scheduled to do the insemination. Although I normally went in for insemination by myself and one of the women did it, I wanted Jeff to go with me this time. There was something a little too intimate for me in having a strange man inseminate me. I always had them make sure that the vial of sperm, which was delivered in a styrofoam box to keep it warm and alive, had Jeff's name on it. And I always had to ask the count, because Jeff never grew tired of hearing the fantastical numbers he produced. This time the count was ninety million, which he took great pride in, as if it were some personal best. He liked to regale me with funny stories of beating off in his coat and tie with his pants dropped in the exam room across the hall, looking at one of the dirty magazines they kept on hand. I tried to imagine how he could catch the ejaculate in the little jar provided. He told me he always tapped to get the last million or so out. One day, he said, some flew up and landed on the examining table. He said he had considered leaving it there for the next guy.

Dr. Campbell was bald and nice, a more lighthearted man than Dr. Kuneck. Jeff and I quizzed him quite a bit as I was getting inseminated. We were a bottomless pit of need for answers and reassurances. My own question was none too subtle: Have you actually seen any Pergonal babies? He looked at me in surprise. Of course, he said. I've seen lots of Pergonal babies. There were two flower arrangements on the reception counter, and I asked Linda when I went out if either of them were Pergonal babies. Yes, she said. So there *was* still a chance.

One day at the hospital I ran into Dr. Kuneck in the hall. I didn't always see him. I had my routine checks with Patty and Sandy. I always liked to see Dr. Kuneck, and we stopped to chat. He had been reading my chart, he told me, and I thought, how romantic! He knows my little ways, my fluctuations in temperature, my developing follicles, my estradiol numbers. He's like a god, I thought as I walked away, knowing that it wasn't true. I just wanted it to be. I wanted him to make me pregnant. He was supposed to have that power, wasn't he? I thought about how serious he always looked, and I felt a little maternal toward him. What a huge load he was carrying around, all the hopes and sorrows of all those infertile people. No wonder he looked so somber.

Jeff would go off to work in the morning, and then I'd be alone at home. The house was so silent—something that at times I valued. But now it seemed devoid of all life, including my own. I had arrived in some distant, barren, wintry place. I saw people all around me in their cozy homes, happy, innocent, I felt, while I was living on the dark side of the moon.

I turned down social invitations whenever I could get away with it. I wanted to be alone. I found the effort of being social and convivial a great demand. I saw that I was in danger, that I could become a withdrawn, depressed, sad person. I felt locked into a strange kind of inertia, where I didn't want to do a thing, literally a thing. I lay in bed, often in the afternoons, with the blinds drawn, the phone machine on. It was like a suspension—a waiting—a kind of concentration that was more physical than mental. I was still passing, on the surface, but my deepest desire was to burrow.

I went in for the next round of insemination by myself. I was feeling very low. I tried not to hide these feelings too much from Debby, a new nurse whom I was getting to know. I thought if there was one place where I could show my true feelings, it was at the infertility clinic. We talked along as she did the insemination. I always enjoyed talking to Debby; she made me think of cool, clear water. She was kind, sympathetic, and as soon as I expressed some of my feelings I felt a little better. Gradually, we began to talk about clothes. We tended to wear similar things, comfortable cotton things that were stylish but not too. She cranked up the bed so that my hips were up in the air, to keep the sperm from running out, and stayed on a while to chat with me. We talked about our endless quest to find some comfortable alternative to pantyhose; she shared my disgust with them, how they "cut you in two." She was wearing knee-high socks under her long skirt, and asked if I had tried thigh-highs. I hadn't in years. She said hers fell down around her ankles on Nicollet Mall, and I told her of dropping out shoulder pads here and there. I thought how much I liked her, how much I liked women. It had helped to have this simple conversation, to make this small connection.

I had to go down to the hospital pharmacy to buy the next round of Pergonal. The pharmacist made a big loud deal over how I shouldn't leave the Pergonal in the car, because it could freeze. It was about a thousand dollars worth of drugs. I felt that all the people around me knew my business: I was forty-two years old, personally responsible for the inflation in health insurance rates, hopelessly trying to get pregnant when it was too late, and worst of all, coming to the end.

As I was leaving I saw a woman ahead of me in the corridor who reminded me of Mother. She was small, stoop-shouldered with age and care. Her hair was the same pale champagne color as Mother's, with the same bald spot in back where she slept on it. At the sight of her a poignancy overcame me. And then I realized that walking with her was another woman, her daughter, I supposed—a middle-aged woman who would, of course, be me.

19

We had a conference with Dr. Kuneck and the verdict seemed to be that it was about over for us. We asked him about the GIFT program, but he had just gotten the latest national statistics for women over forty in such programs; the success rate was 9 percent. And my potential for miscarriage if I did get pregnant was 40 percent. Age was the biological wall and I had my back to it. He said my estradiol numbers were low. Some of the eggs just weren't able to do more. That made Jeff feel sorry for them—"as if we're asking them to do something they can't do," he said sadly. We could try three more rounds of Pergonal, but he thought maybe forty-two was the cutoff point.

It was difficult for me to return each time to the infertility clinic now. The realization that I was counting down to the end was tough. I couldn't imagine not going to the hospital anymore, not seeing the people there, not trying.

I was feeling so isolated that I got the idea of forming a support group of women over forty who were patients at the infertility clinic. I thought such women were different from women in their twenties and thirties. I figured that, like me, women over forty must be having to face an age-related end. We might be able to help each other along in that process.

Dr. Kuneck and Dr. Campbell were very amenable to the idea. They readily agreed to have Linda mail copies of a letter I had written to all their women patients over forty. I included my name and phone number, and told them to give me a call if they were interested in being in a support group.

I dropped off the letter the next time I went in for insemination. I had two good follicles developing, and Dr. Campbell did the insemination. He commented, concerning my effort to get a support group together, that men would never do that. "There's something about that Y chromosome," he joked.

On the way home from the insemination, I thought to myself, I'm going to get pregnant—why shouldn't I? I was surrounded by naysayers (not the least of whom was myself), but why couldn't it work? Why wouldn't it work out? I didn't see why it shouldn't. Why shouldn't I have a baby if I wanted one? Why not me? I hadn't given up hope yet. Hope couldn't be killed off. It was like a worm that someone chops up over and over with a hoe, and still pieces of it live. It couldn't be killed off, hope. It wiggled away, a tiny piece of it, to live on its own.

It was hard to imagine now what the hope was

even for. A baby. A pregnancy. At a certain point it all had become a bit abstract, almost meaningless. I was just engaged in *trying*. I hated to be defeated. I hated to say uncle. I squirmed like a piece of worm meat trying to get away from the hoe.

How had having a baby, getting pregnant, become such an obsession with me? All I could think was that there must be a mechanism that clicks in once you try to get pregnant that instead of allowing you to accept that you cannot, compels you to keep trying, no matter what the odds or cost. Maybe it was actually a biological response, something built in at the deepest level to ensure the species would go on. I had never seen anything like it myself. I never would have suspected, until I tapped into it, just how powerful the desire could be.

And yet I was eventually going to have to quit. I even wanted to quit. But I didn't know how. Did I have to be dead to quit? Sometimes I felt that if allowed, I would just keep on and on, never accepting it as long as I lived. I had seen a headline in the *National Enquirer* one day in the grocery line, "101-Year Old Woman Gives Birth." My immediate thought was that she must have been in infertility treatment and just kept on until she finally succeeded.

I had never imagined, when I was a little girl growing up in South Carolina, that one day I'd be forty-two years old, living in Minnesota, and sitting around with a group of other women over forty feeling envious because I didn't have as many follicles as someone else. There were ten women at the first meeting of the over-forty support group, and we started with our reproductive histories. Marcy, forty-five, a tall Scandinavian looking blond with bangs, had had her first baby at fifteen and given it up for adoption. She had married in her thirties and had had six pregnancies since, none of which had made it to term.

Gina, who wore her dark hair in a long braid down her back, was forty-one and recovering from a laparoscopy that had removed massive fibroids from her uterus. "I'm planning to try in vitro six times," she said. "Do you want to see my scar?" and she pulled down her slacks to show us. She had had two abortions when she was young, before she married. In addition to her fibroid problem, her husband had a low sperm count, so they were having to use frozen donor sperm.

Dede, a pert redhead who was about a size three, had tried GIFT once, and was preparing to try again. "Dr. Kuneck told me I have the ovaries of a thirty-year-old," she said proudly. Someone asked her her estradiol numbers. "I'm producing around fourteen follicles each cycle on Clomid," Dede said, "and my estradiol is right up there around fourteen hundred." I could barely produce two follicles, and my estradiol struggled to get to five hundred.

But then there was Terry, who was just forty (so young!), but who had been trying for ten years unsuccessfully. "I'm not producing any eggs, even on Pergonal," she said sadly. "Dr. Kuneck wants me to quit, but I don't want to. I'm just not ready yet."

"You don't have to," Dede said forcefully. "It's your decision. Just remain positive."

"That's easy for you to say," one of the women shot at Dede. "You've got the ovaries of a thirty-year-old!"

We all laughed, but I saw that Terry was near to tears. Several of the other women already had children, from previous or current marriages, and couldn't conceive or carry another pregnancy to term. "People don't understand about secondary in-fertility," Louise, the mother of an eight-year-old, said. "If you want another child, and can't have one, it's still a big loss. My own mother is always saying to me, 'You've got Kerry, why can't you just be happy.'"

The patient whom Dr. Kuneck had mentioned to me who was forty-eight was there, only now she was forty-nine. "I just didn't get the urge to have a child," she explained, "until I was forty-seven." I felt glad to be among these women, more interested than I would ever have believed in their stories.

But I woke in the middle of the night, troubled by it all. Dede, the one with the ovaries of a thirty-year-old, was a very strong, forceful personality, and she had dominated the group. The message she gave out was that any effort was worth it, that if we'd just be gung ho, we'd succeed. Maybe it was easier to be upbeat if you were producing double-digit follicles each cycle on Pergonal. But most of those women were struggling to make one follicle. One of them was taking four thousand dollars worth of fertility drugs a month to produce one follicle and ending up ovulating early on day twenty-six. It occurred to me now, deep in the night, that some of those women were even further into denial than I was. I thought that none of them, with the possible exception of Dede, had more than a 1–10 percent chance. But they wanted, so it appeared, to keep on. I had never felt my chances were less than 20 percent, but now, after meeting the other women over forty, I felt that maybe they were actually less than that. I suspected that none of those women was going to get pregnant and have a live birth. Of course I could be wrong—that was the problem. We were always hearing success stories, of women over forty who had "miracle" births. But for most of us, I saw, that was not going to happen, and it was disturbing to me that we would all persist so.

At one point in the evening I had said, "It's got to be all right for women not to have children." They had all said of course it was all right, but it didn't seem all right for them. But maybe the more important question was, *Was it all right for me?* Maybe I should get a grip on myself. I, who had always wanted to be in control, had actually lost control of my life. Seeing those infertility patients over forty, I had the uneasy feeling that we were all seriously unbalanced. I didn't think it was unnatural to want a child. I wanted one myself. But I did question pursuing such an unlikely goal in the twilight of our fertility. Was it worth it to wreck our lives emotionally and financially? Weren't we just postponing the inevitable? Was the need for a child so powerful that it swept away rational thought? I couldn't judge the other women. But what did it say about me that I had let the desire for a child take over my life? Didn't I have enough sense of self by this time, enough maturity, really, to accept—even embrace— my life as it was? If I couldn't have a baby, was I going to become a baby myself?

Still, I understood too well how hard it was to give up. Even as I lay there calculating my own long odds, I hoped that I was pregnant. I was in the waiting state again; my period wasn't due until spring break, when we would be in Greenville.

I had made an appointment in Greenville with another infertility specialist for a second opinion. My mother had sent me a news clipping about a doctor in town who had written several articles on infertility. I called his office and told his nurse that I wanted to make an appointment for a consultation. I wanted another opinion on whether or not it was too late.

Jeff was a little skeptical of this idea. But he was willing for me to do whatever I needed to do. I knew I already had all the information and answers I needed. So it wasn't answers and information I was after. It was something else. What if Dr. Kuneck was wrong? What if he was a certain type of personality, very conservative, who himself gave up too soon? I needed to hear it from someone else, to be sure. I was looking for reassurance that it *was* too late. I felt that if I heard it again, from someone else, it would make it easier to end. But I also wanted, I realized, the possibility of some salvation, as if another doctor might say, miraculously, it's certainly not too late! You still have a good chance!

We were in Greenville and it was the thirty-first day of my cycle. Tomorrow, I'd have the appointment with the specialist to get a second opinion. I had not concerned myself too much with starting my period. I was not going to be suckered again. I usually started my period on day thirty-one on Pergonal, so I hadn't given it much thought until day thirty. Then I thought, simply, Well, I'll just start tomorrow. And that will be the end of that.

All day on the thirty-first day, I waited for my period. It was going to come. I felt bloated, crampy. Still, it didn't come and it didn't come. By evening, I was beginning to allow myself the thought that I might be pregnant. My mind seized the smallest possibility and ran with it. Soon I was actually delivering, a live birth as they say in the statistics I'd become so familiar with. All through the night, I tossed and turned, I got up to see if I had started my period and I hadn't. It was agony. Could I really be pregnant? At last? And might it not work out this time? It might . . . I imagined the irony of going in to the infertility specialist tomorrow and asking for a pregnancy test. I imagined calling back to my clinic in Minneapolis, to tell them the amazing news. I burned all night long with fears and hopes, knowing I was probably not pregnant, but unable to let go of the possibility. It was a feverish, nightmarish, anguishing night. When I got up in the morning, day thirty-two, my period had arrived.

I didn't know it at the time, but it would never be like that for me again. I would never allow myself to go through another night like that one. It went too far. They had played with me enough, finally. They had made me suffer a little too much that time. I didn't even know it, but I was about to cut them off, those devils of hope and despair.

Jeff and I went to see the infertility specialist. He was a bit disorganized. When he began talking with us, I realized he had not read my files, which I had been so diligent in having sent down ahead of time. He seemed to want to figure out what was wrong with me, why I couldn't get pregnant, but I told him I had been completely checked out, it was all in my records. He seemed to want to second-guess Dr. Kuneck, and I thought I detected some male competition at work. I felt like telling him what was wrong with me was my age. As Jeff would say later, did we really have to pay a hundred and twenty-five dollars to find that out?

"It takes a woman over forty about eighteen cycles to get pregnant," he told us. He was a bald man in his fifties, in a navy blue jacket with gold nautical buttons. He reminded me of certain Southern men I had seen all my life, the country club set, the mint julep type, confident and cocky within a small local pond. "Of course, Pergonal ups those chances somewhat, but you can't stay on Pergonal forever. I'd back away from Pergonal," he said. "I'd back away from artificial insemination. There is always a chance, after all, until you hit menopause."

I was shocked. Not using artificial insemination was in direct contradiction to what Dr. Kuneck thought improved our chances. There was obviously a difference of opinion here.

"But I thought artificial insemination improved the chances of conceiving," I said.

"Nonsense," he said, rocking back in his desk chair. "In fact, it might hinder conception. Timing isn't all that important. You should just do the natural thing. You'll naturally become," he said looking at me, "the sexual aggressor a few days before ovulation." Jeff and I raised our eyebrows at each other. The guy had obviously never been in infertility treatment himself.

When we left Jeff shook his head. "What a hustler," he said animatedly. "He obviously wants you for a patient. And what was that about wanting to give you a physical? The guy gave me the creeps!"

I had to laugh. I didn't know myself if he were a hustler or a creep, and I didn't really care. I had gotten what I had come for. I was looking for some kind of loophole, some way to stop without hitting the wall. Rational thought aside, I knew I wasn't ready for The End. He had said he'd back off Pergonal; he'd back off artificial insemination. I wanted to back off of all that. He had said we could still keep trying, the natural way. The message I had heard was that we could stop infertility treatment, but that we still had a chance. We had a small chance right up until menopause, and that let me off the hook, the horrible hook that it was completely over.

We enjoyed being with my parents. I was able to do things to help them out, such as take my mother to the doctor, and drive my father to the barber shop, since he couldn't drive himself anymore. At eighty-seven he was having more and more trouble with his short-term memory, but he was as pleasant as always to be with. I'd see him dozing in the La-Z-Boy rocker, and he reminded me of an old dog or cat, sleeping in the peace and comfort of old age. Nothing much disturbed him. He was very attached to my mother, who looked after him now that he couldn't quite look after himself. When she drove to the beauty parlor one day, he rushed to the front window, and watched her back out of the driveway and turn onto Jones Street. He wanted to make sure she made it safely into the street. When they went somewhere, my mother told me, he always had to keep her in sight. In his old age my father was becoming a bit of a child himself again.

One night Jeff, Mother, and I played three-handed bridge. All four of us had had a good time before dinner watching the news and having cocktails, cheese, and crackers, green pepper jelly over cream cheese, and cocktail wienics with hot sauce. My parents loved a good cocktail hour, and so did we. My father never played bridge, so after dinner my mother and I tried to teach Jeff. We sat in the living room on the needlepoint dining room chairs at a card table. Jeff found a piece of old chewing gum stuck to the bottom of his chair, which he promptly displayed. He teased my mother about which of her bridge-playing friends stuck gum under her chair. We were all laughing, having a good time, and I felt more relaxed, I realized, than I had in a long time. For a moment at least life was not some monumental problem to solve, there were no hard decisions to make, no hard realities to face, no grief or pain, just a three-handed bridge game with my mother and Jeff and a piece of old gum stuck under a chair.

That night I had the "provided for" dream. In the dream I was struggling. A lot of people were going to show up at our cabin, and I was going to have to feed them all. But when they arrived, they were all carrying food. I didn't have to do anything; it was being taken care of. The people were from all different parts of my life, time ran together, the past and the present were one.

Aunt Grace and Uncle Perry came over before we left. Two years ago they had moved to a retirement home and they were finally making the adjustment. They looked frail in their old age, but they were alive, they were still themselves. I hugged my mother good-bye in the house, and then Daddy, along with Aunt Grace and Uncle Perry, who were driving us to the airport, went out with us to the car. I hugged my father good-bye. March 18, 1990. I felt how small he was. I felt his bony loving hands on my back. I smelled the skin of his face. Good-bye, Daddy, good-bye. I climbed into the car, and as we were pulling down the driveway, I turned to see him once more. He stood watching us go.

We flew on to Florida, to see Jeff's parents who were wintering there. One morning before we were to leave, I woke up early. Jeff was still sleeping, and I looked across to the twin bed where he lay on blue sheets, beautiful in the early light. It came to me that it really was a choice between two good things—having a child and not having a child. Our life without a child seemed good to me. I caught a glimpse that it was what was right for us, for the best. But who can say what is "best"? Maybe it's possible to get to a place where what is best is simply *what is*.

20

Any equilibrium I had gained in South Carolina and Florida flew out the door when I returned to Minneapolis. Back in my own life, I still had the problem of letting go. I knew I was at the end, but I still couldn't end it. The pain of never having a child seemed to me so enormous that I couldn't look it in the face.

I had never really considered adoption; I had been fixated on having a biological child. But the fact that adoption was one way of ending the pain was brought home to me when a couple we knew called to say that they had just adopted a baby. That proved to me that people could get babies, which was different from infertility.

I had begun to think that we would be all right if we didn't have a child, but our friends' adopting threw me into new turmoil. Maybe I was only coming to the end of infertility, and once I resolved that, we would move on to adoption. I knew that was an option. But I wasn't sure it was one that I wanted to pursue. Trying to have a child had dominated my life for several years, and I felt emotionally tired of it all. I was almost forty-three years old, and I wanted to be through. I had run out of energy for wanting a child. I believed, rationally, that I could be all right without a child. But I wasn't sure I could get through the pain without adopting.

I went to another meeting of the fortysomething group, where the talk turned to adoption. One woman had been actively pursuing adoption in Chile, but now things were getting more restricted there, and the adoption she had thought she had arranged had fallen through. They would have had to fly to Chile and stay several months. The cost would be between five thousand and ten thousand dollars. There was talk of other countries where older couples could adopt.

Adoption was clearly an option. I could make it right by adopting, I could get a child, I could be a mother. But I wasn't the same person I had been when I had first embarked on this reproduction odyssey. I had to reassess again now. I knew that for me, adoption would be another long-drawn-out emotional process. It would probably take several years.

And I had to admit that I was somewhat afraid of adoption. I was uncertain about the child I might get—a complete unknown. I didn't believe each child was a blank slate on which loving parents could write whatever they wished. I believed in nature as well as nurture, in genes, heredity. That didn't mean that we shouldn't adopt. A biological child, after all, was also an unknown. But someone else's genes seemed a bigger unknown.

It did trouble me that we were capable of providing a loving, stable home to a child who needed one, and that we weren't going to. I figured that many people who adopted didn't do so out of pure altruism, but rather to satisfy their own needs, to parent, to nurture and love unconditionally, and also to "fit in," be part of the human experience. But I felt the "selfish" finger would be pointed at me for not adopting; I would point it, to some extent, myself.

I called Dr. Kuneck and left a message for him to call me. I hadn't started another round of Pergonal since returning from Florida and now I wanted to tell him I was through. He returned my call at ten on a Sunday night, taking me by surprise. He had been so busy, he apologized, that he hadn't been able to return my call until now.

"Well," I began slowly, "I won't be back for any more treatment. I've been giving it a lot of thought, and I don't think it's the best thing now for me to continue on this course."

"I understand," he said thoughtfully. "That makes sense."

"We're just going to take our chances," I said. "We're not going to use birth control, but I don't really expect to get pregnant."

"I'd say your chances are about 5 percent," he

said, "though of course I really don't know." We were both silent for a moment. "We could give you a test to see how well you're ovulating off Pergonal, if you want."

"No. No more tests."

"I think you've conducted yourself with intelligence and logic all through this," he said.

I thanked him and we said our good-byes. I felt proud of myself, discussing the end so calmly and rationally. But as soon as I hung up—*as soon as he was gone!*—I began to weep.

Jeff and I decided to go to an orientation meeting of an independent adoption agency. I wanted to make sure we didn't want to adopt. I knew that a lot of people who went through infertility eventually adopted, after they had mourned the loss of a biological child. I wondered if that was what was in store for us. Jeff wasn't particularly interested in adopting. But he was willing if that was what I wanted to do. We could borrow the money, or take out a loan. We agreed that money was a factor, but that it wasn't the main consideration. If we wanted to adopt, there were ways.

At the meeting there was a lot of information about birth mothers, mostly young girls living in rural Minnesota who had gotten pregnant and now wanted to give their babies up for adoption. Most of the other people there were older couples like us who weren't able to have children on their own. If we joined up, we were told, we would be taught how to write a letter to attract a young pregnant woman's attention. I didn't want to write a letter to attract a young pregnant woman's attention. I knew we'd never go any further than this, the orientation meeting.

I decided not to go to the next meeting of the fortysomething group. I decided I was no longer appropriate. I was at the end, and the group was for people who wanted to keep on. I wondered if maybe I had created a monster. I had meant the group to be a place where women could resolve the issue, come to closure, but it seemed a vehicle for keeping people going. Maybe that was fine. I wished them well, but I was no longer one of them.

It was the end of March, and I wanted winter to be over. If only spring would come! I uncovered my garden, raking off the straw, feeling cold and lonely. The next day I had to cover everything up again, because the forecast was for a hard freeze.

I hadn't been to church in years, but now I started visiting different churches. I wanted to be in a sacred place, and I wanted to hear someone speak of God's way, God's knowing, as opposed to human knowledge, or more specifically, my knowledge. In one church I visited, before the service people got up and lit slender tapers. I was moved by these people, touched by whatever grief or loss was in their hearts. I would have liked to go up and light a candle myself, but I was afraid to. I was afraid I'd break down.

I talked to my mother every week on the phone. One Sunday when she first recognized my voice, she said, "Hi, doll," and I felt warmed, nurtured. When I told her, shakily, that I had about decided not to have a child, she said, "Paulette, I've been giving this a lot of thought. And I think you're right. I think it really isn't the best thing, now, for you to take on a child. I think you're going to be fine. I want you to get on with your life—with loving Jeff, with writing." When I hung up, the tears flowed again. My mother had helped release me.

Then it was May, and I was forty-three years old.

I had lunch one day with another writer in town who I knew had adopted a child. I wanted to know about her experience with adoption. I was still troubled that perhaps I was making a mistake in not adopting.

"I've had to back into every major decision of my life," Jane told me in her calm, quiet way. "I didn't get married until I was thirty-five, and then when I actually started thinking about having a child, my main feelings were ambivalence and hysteria."

"Ambivalence I understand," I said. "But why hysteria?"

"Hysteria that it might already be too late."

I nodded.

"My husband didn't want children, or at least he didn't then. But I got pregnant right away. I lost that one at four months. Then I got pregnant again and lost that one at six months. Meantime we were looking into adoption, and suddenly, we got a Korean baby." Tears filled her eyes. "All the questions about adoption—who is this child, where does he come from—didn't matter to me then, because he arrived alive, and I was used to children not arriving alive." Now tears flooded my eyes.

"How has motherhood been for you?"

"It hasn't really changed my life all that much, or kept me from writing," she said. "But having a child is a challenge and a lot of work."

"I don't know if I can get over the pain without adopting," I said.

"Unless you resolve it. Unless it is over. Unless you get out of this state of wondering if you're going to adopt and make the decision not to. Then you might be at peace."

I appreciated Jane telling me her story, talking to me about her experience. She was balancing her life, having her baby and writing, and that was right for her. She didn't make motherhood out to be something mystical or irresistible. I didn't feel any pressure coming from her about what I should do. Still, I felt in my heart, for reasons I couldn't really fathom, that what was right for her wasn't right for me.

But what a decision to make! I could end the pain I was feeling, I could adopt, I could have a child, and yet I wasn't going to. An inner sense told me that what I needed to do was get through this, that there would be life beyond—my life. But I wasn't sure I could do it. Giving up on a child felt like a death. It was a death, but there was no ritual, no ceremony to mark it. There was no body, no funeral.

A friend had told me about a psychic she had gone to see, so I made an appointment as a birthday gift to myself. I was searching for a sign that the decision I was making — *never to have a child* — was in accordance with my true self. I was feeling my way in the dark, aware that I was engaged in a process that was beyond my control, but which nevertheless I had to trust to get me through.

I had never been to a psychic before, which was part of the appeal. I wished I could visit a shaman, a seer, a wise elder who could show me the way. I would have liked to go to a hut full of smoke and fire, and have some grizzled old woman speak enigmatically to me of things I knew, but didn't know I knew. If that was asking too much of the psychic, which I suspected it was, at least it might be an interesting experience.

Maureen's house was an attractive brown split-level folded into the bank of a wooded lot in a northern suburb. I parked under some oak trees and went in on the first level. Maureen answered the door, accompanied by an overweight golden retriever. She was maybe five years younger than I, thin with a chiseled face and dark red hair. She wasn't wearing any makeup, had on cutoff blue jeans and a T-shirt, and was barefoot. We smiled warmly at each other, ready to like one another. She led me upstairs to the living room, which was light and airy. No campfire, not even a candle, but there was a big picture window, and a nice deck out back with a Weber grill.

Maureen led me to an overstuffed armchair and pulled up a straight back chair in front of me. She loaded a blank tape into her small tape recorder, and explained what type of work she did. She wasn't a fortune teller, she said, and she didn't talk about what might happen in the future. She tried to allow a person access to stuck areas, "to light them up."

When she closed her eyes and began her deep breathing, I closed my eyes, too. I tried to relax, though I felt intense. There was nothing I had to do now. I had gotten myself here, and now I could be silent, still. I was the seeker, the listener. Something had brought me here, to Maureen's, and I sensed that this was the right place to be.

"Say your full name."

My voice sounded thin to me, watery, full of tears.

She shifted around in her chair a bit, concentrating with her eyes shut. "It feels to me like you worry a lot."

I snorted and she opened her eyes. "Do you?"

"Well, a little," I admitted, then added anxiously, "but doesn't everyone?"

She laughed lightly. "Sure." Then she shut her

eyes again. "But with you, the worrying gets things stuck. You keep the problems stuck and unsolved, because of the worrying, rather than letting go and trusting that you'll get the answer. You think if you can think things out, you can bypass the emotions."

She looked at me. "I guess we all want to bypass the feelings sometimes."

She shut her eyes and concentrated again. "Something is stuck here," she said. "Emotions feel scary to you—as if, if you have the emotions, you'll come apart. But it's just the opposite of what you think. It's the *not having* them that will cause you to fall apart."

"I don't exactly feel like a person cut off from her emotions," I said hesitantly. "In fact, most of the time I have too many of them."

"But you have to release them. You're full of emotions because you don't give in to them."

She was still for a moment, eyes shut. She shifted around in her chair. "Don't compare yourself," she said emphatically. "When you compare, you lose yourself. *They* did it right, *I* did it wrong. It's as if you don't trust yourself well enough."

We were both silent for a long moment.

"There's something here," she said. "I'm not sure what the issue is—but part of the conflict is shoulds and shouldn'ts, rights and wrongs, judgments, how things *ought* to be. You have to sweep them all away. They're fueling things so big. If you get rid of all the shoulds and oughts, you'll *know*. The knowing will still be hard, but at least you'll know. Everyone else's energy clouds you from the way *you* want to be."

I could feel something building inside. It hurt my chest.

"You need to take the right and wrong out of it," Maureen said. "There is no right or wrong here. Only what feels correct for you in your life."

I wanted to give up on having a child! I wanted to be able to walk away from that and know that I would be all right—but I wasn't sure I could. *How could it possibly be right if it was so painful?*

"Even if it's painful?" I asked in a choked voice.

"Even if it's painful," Maureen said firmly. *"Some of our best decisions are our most painful ones."*

Something cracked open inside me, maybe my heart. It cracked like a crockery plate. Tears flooded my eyes.

"Are you all right?" Maureen asked quietly.

I was too full and empty to speak.

I was wiping away the tears.

"Do you want to talk about it?" Maureen asked gently.

I told her about trying to get pregnant, trying to decide about adoption, trying to accept that I was giving up on having a child.

"My sense is that the pain and grief keep sending you back. Because to give that up—it's so sad!"

"Yes, it is!" I wept again. "It's *so* sad!"

"It's like having to know who you are without

that part of yourself. The part that other women have. It's hard to accept your own decision—*How could I not do it?*"

She paused to consider. "But what are your goals in this lifetime? You have to look at that."

We were both silent again.

"There is a true ache in the body to walk away from it," she said solemnly. "A true ache, until it is accepted and resolved. We were made to have babies. There's nothing more to it than that. Our bodies were made to have babies, and it takes a long time for the body to get over not having them.

"But the ache does go away," she said. "It does let up."

We were both silent.

"Once you walk through the grief—once you resolve it—I think there will be a lot of relief."

We had taken a break, and now Maureen was smoking a cigarette. "I know what you're feeling," she said when I sat back down, "because I went through the same thing myself."

I stared at her. "About having a child?" Then I thought of what I had known all along, without even thinking of it. No children lived here.

"That's right," Maureen said. "The whole nine yards. So I know what you're going through. It was very, very painful for me. I couldn't even stand to see a baby. I couldn't go in a room with a baby. It's an *agony*, and no one understands that."

"But . . . what about now?"

"Now, the only thing is just sometimes wondering what it would have been like to have a kid," she said calmly. "Because it's an incredible thing to do! But it didn't fit in my life. I didn't know that at the time. But now I think, what if we had kids running around here!" She laughed in her deep voice. "My whole life would have to change. I know now that wasn't right for me."

I considered this for a while. "I don't meet many women who've resolved this by not having children," I said.

She nodded. "Do you have any other things you want to talk about?"

I told her I had gotten what I had come for.

"Then the final thing I'd say to you is do what's right for you—whether anyone else gets it or not. Then you will be at peace. Learn to trust yourself. You have to practice what feels right for you. This whole crisis has been about learning who *you* are. Where you have trouble is in not believing that you know. But you do know. You know.

Driving home, I knew it was over. *Some of our best choices are our most painful ones*. I believed in trying to make the right choices in my life. Maybe our lives are really just little boats of rationalization floating on an ocean of unconscious values, circumstances, conditioning, and needs beyond our control. Still, I thought it was worth the effort to at least maintain the illusion that one was steering the boat.

But the knowing that takes place in our heads is

a lot different from the knowing that takes place in our hearts. There's the rational and the emotional, the decision and the grief. Some of our best choices are our most painful ones.

That evening, telling Jeff about my visit with Maureen, I began to sob. I sobbed into Jeff's chest, and I didn't try to stop. *I wasn't going to have a child. I was never going to have a child!* I dissolved into grief. I became Grief itself. *I was never going to have a child.*

It felt as if I were going to die. But I didn't die. It was crying, not dying. And it was a great relief.

Later that night, we went out for Chinese food. I was drained, but true to form, also hungry. I felt lighter than I had felt in a long time—peaceful, as if I had returned from a long, difficult journey. The fortune in my fortune cookie read, "You are almost there."

Coda

It was Gertrude Stein who said there is no there there (she was referring to Oakland). But regarding the pain of never having a child, I'd have to say there is no there there, either. It's not as if you arrive at some place (Oakland or otherwise) where you no longer feel it. Where you're *over* it. It's the same as with any loss. You take it into your body; it becomes a part of you. But Maureen was right: the ache does go away.

There are moments, however, when I still feel the loss. Take the other night, for example. We were at that same Chinese restaurant, only this time with Jeff's brother Peter and his wife, Mary Ellen, and their two children, Maggie and John. The occasion was John's birthday, and Uncle Jeff and I were happy to be included. Earlier, we had gone to the Zoo Store to buy presents for the children. On the floor of the store was a quacking, honking, roaring, roving menagerie of animals, all battery activated. For Maggie we bought the pink pig that rotated its snout, wiggled its curlicue tail, and oinked; for John, the gray hippo that roared with a wide pink mouth. At home Jeff put batteries in, and the pig and hippo waddled across our dining room rug. We were both laughing, and I thought of how much fun it would be to have children of our own. I didn't feel particularly sad, the way I might have once. I was just aware of what we were missing.

And there did come a moment at the table when I felt a real pang. Maggie had climbed into Mary Ellen's lap after dinner and wrapped her arms around her neck. I glanced over to see Mary Ellen nuzzling her child's head, burying her face into the fine blond hair, smelling that sweet child smell. I had to look away then. But in a little while I looked back, to witness such a beautiful sight.

On the way home I asked Jeff how he felt about not having children. "Well, I feel regret," he said, "but having children is something I didn't get in my life. I can't spend the rest of my life feeling bad about it."

I understood what he meant. Having children was something we didn't get. A certain amount of luck is involved. Life doesn't always give you what you expect or want, though it may give you different, possibly better things.

I used to imagine a shadow self, a woman who was another version of me. She had stayed on in Greenville, married a doctor, had children, and whirled around town in a station wagon, chauffeuring everybody to dentist appointments, piano lessons, Girl Scouts—just as my mother had done. Even though I knew better, it seemed to some part of me that this shadow self was leading the "correct" life, the life I should have been leading. For a long time it kept me from accepting my own, real life, in Minnesota, being a writer, not having children.

Somewhere along the way, that shadow self died. I realized I was not her, could never have been her. I'm in the midst of my own life, and if it isn't the life I might have expected exactly, it is the life I have. I tend to think it's the life I've wanted, in spite of myself. I happen to like it. It seems to me a rich and blessed life. Every day I'm grateful for it.

I go back to Greenville about twice a year. There's only my mother and Aunt Grace now. My father died on September 2, 1990, of a heart attack, at the age of eighty-seven. And while I never would have been ready to lose him, I'm glad he waited as long as he did for me to grow up. It's only in the last year or so that I've felt my own maturity somewhat in place.

Uncle Perry died on April 17, 1992, of congestive heart failure. I made it to Greenville in time to say good-bye; he died exactly an hour after I arrived at the hospital.

Mr. Stegner has died too, at age eighty-four, of injuries suffered in a car accident.

How I miss those fathers!

My mother has aged quite a bit since my father died. She can barely walk, the result of arthritis and several falls. But she wants to stay on in her own home as long as she can. Betty and I take turns going there to see about her. It makes me sad that she is alone now so much of the time.

As for Aunt Grace, she lives alone in the retirement home, almost blind from macular degeneration and cataracts. She's frail but resilient, it appears.

Often I think of the time when both Mother and Aunt Grace will be gone. Then Greenville, at least for me, will be gone, too. I'll still return occasionally, to see friends and cousins, but all the old ones will be gone. So much will be gone!

I still dream about cats. Cats run through my dreams.

Jeff's been a solo attorney long enough now to have learned to roll with the ups and downs of it. On the weekends he's writing a comic novel, something that is giving him enormous pleasure and satisfaction. He's always felt that writing was his best self, but for a long time he had to put it aside. In the past few years he's been able to reclaim that part of himself.

I suppose by some people's standards we're a bit odd. Most Saturdays find us sitting a wall apart, him in the guest room at a desk he put together from a kit, me in my study at my uncle Perry's old rolltop desk I had shipped up from South Carolina, both of us writing. We're both interested in writing and books. We're carrying on an extended conversation we began nearly twenty years ago, and neither of us has grown tired of it.

Sunday mornings usually find us back in bed

after breakfast. Those are sweet times—making love, and then some extra sleep, delicious when it's cold and snowy outside, which, let's face it, it often is in Minnesota. Because we don't have children around, we're able to pay all the more attention to each other. I suppose there is some danger in that—that we'll become too attached, or too insular or too—something. But I have to say I feel lucky for what we have.

I'm teaching at a small liberal arts college now. I'm pleased to help the students, who teeter between childhood and adulthood, with their writing—with all that writing can do for them. I find I have a lot of patience. I take the long view.

I've been teaching two courses this term, creative writing and freshman English, as I can't seem to get over calling it, though I ought to say "college English" or "composition," and refer to the students as "first-year," not freshmen. The irony is that in class we had a big discussion about gender-biased terms, and I had to be the defender of using terms like "humankind" instead of "mankind." It wasn't a burning issue with me, but someone had to remind them of the time when everyone took it for granted that the pronoun "he" could stand for all of us. It disturbed me to hear my students pooh-pooh feminism as they did. "Those feminists," several of them said, distancing themselves from the enemy.

Recently I went over an essay with one of the young women in the class. The assignment for the paper had been "proposing a solution." The students were supposed to come up with a problem and then figure out the means to alleviate it. World hunger. The food at the campus cafeteria. This young woman had written about premarital sex. It had taken me a minute to grasp what the problem was. Too much of it. The fact that it existed at all. STD, AIDS. The solution was to save yourself for marriage. For a moment I felt I was back in the fifties; but of course we're in the nineties now. The student, serious, smart, and unhappy looking, believed that she'd regret it if she had sex before marriage. I went over the paper, making suggestions regarding organization and wording, keeping to myself my own premarital history. I contemplated this young woman, who could have been my daughter, with a certain amount of bemusement. What differences would the trials and errors of my generation of women make in her choices in life? Would she be spared some of the conflicts, confusions, and trade-offs of my own female life? How would the beliefs she was formulating now, when she was so young, influence the course of her life for the next twenty years or more? Would things work out for her the way they were "supposed" to? I had no answers to these questions. But I wished her well with all my heart.

A while back I was asked to be on an "Alternatives" panel at a Hoping and Coping Conference—a "one day seminar for individuals and couples dealing with the stresses of infertility." I roped Jeff into appearing with me, although I had to pay a price—he immediately began referring to it as the "Hoping and Moping" conference. He wasn't really mean-hearted, it was just that he couldn't resist a verbal joke, and he felt some lingering resentment toward the world of infertility. We would be the couple on the panel who had resolved infertility by not adopting. When the brochure arrived, I was a little taken aback to see us listed as the "childfree" couple. It brought to mind other "free" words—debt-free, drug-free, carefree. But at least it was better than "childless." There really isn't a word for what we are; just ourselves.

I agreed to be on the panel because I thought it was important for people to hear from others who had survived infertility and who were okay without a child. It's an alternative that doesn't get much play. And I wanted to hear what Jeff and I would say. I myself, as it turns out, need models, even if I have to provide them. I sometimes feel that everyone has children—and those who don't have nothing to say. But for me, not having a child has turned out to be a big experience—perhaps the defining one of my life.

As I began to think about what I wanted to say on the panel, I realized that I wouldn't be able to explain myself fully. I wanted to tell my story and have it make sense to people (and to me). I didn't want to have to simplify it. I thought of a T-shirt I had seen one time in a store window. It had a pic-

ture of a woman with a weeping face and underneath the caption, "Oh no! I forgot to have a baby!"
I had had to laugh, even as it stung. Though I had
had my share of tears, I didn't want to be reduced to
a one-liner. I knew my own experience to be more
complex than that. It occurred to me that it might
be interesting. Well, it interested me.

But I knew that a panel was no place to get into
the complexities of one's life experience. I'd have to
settle for a few sound bites. Actually, that was the
way I felt about most spoken communication. I
often found talking a little like sitting down to play
Rachmaninoff only to have "Chopsticks" come out.

The other two couples on the panel had solved
the problem of infertility by adopting. We sat in fold-
ing chairs on a stage looking out at an audience of
maybe one hundred people. Seeing those people
who were still struggling with infertility made me
feel like weeping. I felt the most intense sympathy
for them, remembering my own hoping, coping,
moping, and more.

Jeff and I told our story, and then the other couples told of their journeys to arrive at adoption. One
of the women, who was maybe thirty, with a kind
of lovely grace to her, told how she had carried a
pregnancy to seven months, then had a stillbirth,
followed by three more miscarriages, all well along.
Now that they had a child through adoption, they
had the emotional energy, she explained, to try again
to have a biological child. "I want to give birth," she

said, then amended, "I have given birth—but I mean to a live child."

The other couple, in their forties, had been married three years. She had gotten pregnant at thirty-nine, only to miscarry, followed by another miscarriage, and they decided not to escalate her treatments to the next stage. They were clearly elated over their adopted son from China. Both couples offered concrete, tangible solutions to the pain of infertility, happy endings, and I was moved by their stories. I wondered once again if we had made the right "choice." I felt that we had, for us, but that didn't mean I never thought about the path not taken.

The session was opened to questions from the audience, and most of them were directed to the adoptive couples. As Jeff said later, "'Childfree' is a hard sell to an infertility audience." A few people did ask us questions, though being Minnesotans, perhaps they were just being polite. One man addressed us in what I thought was a graceful way as "the family of two." But then a woman asked me a question that took me by surprise. "Since you don't have kids," she said, "what do you do with your time?"

My mind went blank. What *did* I do with my time? Clearly not enough! I just did what I had always done—I taught, wrote, cooked, cleaned up, napped, saw friends and family. I loved to waste time, too. I liked nothing better than to daydream, to garden, to read, to remember. The truth was, I always felt I needed more time. I stuttered out that it really wasn't a problem, but I felt a little abashed. A part of me still felt, I was sorry to see, that if I weren't raising children, I wasn't doing "right."

After the conference, we met Peter and Mary Ellen and their kids at the Mall of America. The Rainforest Restaurant had a two-hour wait for a table, so we struggled through the crowd to a fifties-style diner for dinner. Peter and Mary Ellen often seemed preoccupied and exhausted from the demands of their busy lives and their two young children. They sometimes expressed envy that we have so much time for each other, that we can do what we want, that we travel, that we both like to write. But I also know they wouldn't trade.

After dinner they invited us back to their house, but we declined. Instead, Jeff and I wandered through the mall for a while, feeling release, relief. We agreed it had been a good thing to be on the panel, but that we wouldn't want to do it again. It gave us a lot to talk about, though. I said something about how difficult it is to be different sometimes, but how valuable that can be. Jeff expressed "a sense of mourning" that the natural event of having children hadn't worked out for us. We stopped for coffee at Nordstrom's espresso bar.

"I don't know," I mused, peering into the huge space of the Megamall. "I didn't really get out of that panel experience whatever it was I wanted."

"What were you after?"

"There's just so much I didn't get to explain! Like the chortling part. How sometimes I actually chortle to myself that I don't have children. That I didn't have to do it. That I escaped. It's not my main feeling but it's one of them. But how could I ever explain that in public?"

"You know," Jeff said, "the only way you can really tell your story is to write it."

I looked at him for a long moment. "I was afraid you were going to say that."

The next day I got to my study bright and early. I thought of that woman on the T-shirt with the weeping face. I had been raised to expect and assume motherhood. I had expected and assumed it myself, even as I ignored and resisted it. Why was that? How had I come to be a woman who did not have a child?

I often talked to my writing students about launching their stories. The opening, I told them, is all-important. The first sentences should be like a piece of thread that pulls the whole story after it. I told them they didn't need to start at the very beginning. But when I considered my own story, I wanted to start at the beginning, the very beginning, as in "Once upon a time I was a fertilized egg with two X chromosomes." The fact that I had been born female seemed to me the most important thing.

But I took my own advice. I didn't start at the beginning. I picked up my pen and began to write.